CW00369456

MODERN LIVING, HOLISTIC HEALTH & HERBAL MEDICINE

Improving health & well-being with herbs and lifestyle changes

Yaso Shan

With contributions from Dr. Catherine Whitlock and a
Foreword by Jenny Seagrove

Copyright © 2011 Yaso Shan

ISBN 978-1-60910-639-3

All rights reserved. No part of this publication may be reproduced, stored in a retrieval system, or transmitted in any form or by any means, electronic, mechanical, recording or otherwise, without the prior written permission of the author.

Printed in the United States of America.

BookLocker.com, Inc.
2011

First Edition

DISCLAIMER

This book details the author's personal experiences with and opinions about herbal medicine and holistic healthcare approaches. The author is not a healthcare provider.

The author and publisher are providing this book and its contents on an "as is" basis and make no representations or warranties of any kind with respect to this book or its contents. The author and publisher disclaim all such representations and warranties, including for example warranties of merchantability and healthcare for a particular purpose. In addition, the author and publisher do not represent or warrant that the information accessible via this book is accurate, complete or current.

The statements made about products and services have not been evaluated by the U.S. Food and Drug Administration. They are not intended to diagnose, treat, cure, or prevent any condition or disease. Please consult with your own physician or healthcare specialist regarding the suggestions and recommendations made in this book.

Except as specifically stated in this book, neither the author or publisher, nor any authors, contributors, or other representatives will be liable for damages arising out of or in connection with the use of this book. This is a comprehensive limitation of liability that applies to all damages of any kind, including (without limitation) compensatory; direct, indirect or consequential damages; loss of data, income or profit; loss of or damage to property and claims of third parties.

You understand that this book is not intended as a substitute for consultation with a licensed healthcare practitioner, such as your physician. Before you begin any healthcare program, or change your lifestyle in any way, you will consult your physician or other licensed healthcare practitioner to ensure that you are in good health and that the examples contained in this book will not harm you.

This book provides content related to topics physical and/or mental health issues. As such, use of this book implies your acceptance of this disclaimer.

Dedication

I would like to dedicate this book to all my patients, past and present who have shown much courage and strength in battling their illness and coping with the often distressing symptoms with much dignity and a tremendously positive attitude. Their determination and fortitude during their most difficult times has been a total inspiration to me, as a practitioner and as a healer.

Acknowledgements

~ ~ ~ ~ ~ ~

I express my huge gratitude and thanks to my family for all their help and support during the writing of this book, without which I could not have done it.

A special thank you to my mother for her resilience, wisdom, strength of character, love and much encouragement.

A special thank you also to my wonderful sisters, Saratha and Subo to whom I am utterly indebted for their immense help, professional advice, their unstinting support, and quite simply for being my two best friends.

A special dedication and immense gratitude to my late father for his advice and input; his considerable medical experience generated debate and discussion that has been both informative and invaluable. It has certainly given me a rounded perspective on clinical practice. And a very special thank you to my brother Yoga for all his technical help and assistance.

Last but not least, to Patrick, for his patience, guidance, love and understanding. Thank you for being there, I could not have finished this book without your help, support and commitment to my many projects.

~ ~ ~ ~ ~ ~

A very special thank you to Ian McMillan (former Editor of Mental Health Practice and Learning Disability Practice specialist journals at RCN Publishing Company and latterly the British Journal of Wellbeing at MA Healthcare) for being an influential driver in my career in offering me the scope to broaden my journalistic skills into mainstream medical press. I feel very fortunate and privileged to have had the opportunity to work for you. Thank you for your kindness, professionalism and invaluable advice.

I extend an equally special thank you to Stelyana Spassova at the Brackenbury Natural Health Clinic for having had the faith in my skills to offer the opportunity for me to practise at the Clinic. This broadened my client base and extended my clinical experience. The impact was to develop my expertise and to enhance my portfolio which led to significant interest from international audiences. The support from other staff at the Clinic, Liz, Max and Glynnis was equally tremendous.

~ ~ ~ ~ ~ ~

Additional thanks to the following: Julie Sylvester, Editor for Primary Health Care specialist journal who has always been open to my suggestions for the 'alternative perspective' on things. To the other members of the publishing team at the Royal College of Nursing: Karen Davies and Lindsay Fitzpatrick , thank you both so much for doing such a fabulous job on my articles and to Helen Hyland, thank you for your efficiency and general management of the 'housekeeping'! A heartfelt thank you to my mentor Christine Alder, without whose guidance, advice, support and help I could not keep going and continue with the good work of herbalists in helping so many people. To Jenny Seagrove whose commitment and drive in improving consumer choice is a constant inspiration. To my writing collaborator and colleague, Dr Catherine Whitlock, who is simply bliss to work with, both in the exchange of ideas and concepts and in having a mutual understanding of the need to educate and inform. To my web designer and all things technical Philip Mason; thank you so much for your patience, technical help and the numerous call outs! To my graphic designer Sarah Browne; thank you for all your help with my business design and for your wonderful creativity. To my clinical supervisors David Keogh and Hananja Brice-Ytsma at the Archway Clinical of Herbal Medicine; I learnt so much for you both and I thank you for sharing your knowledge and clinical expertise. To all the staff at the Archway Clinic of Herbal Medicine and the teaching staff at Middlesex University; thank you for the good work you all do in delivering a wonderful service to patients and in providing a great training programme and academic research for future practitioners of herbal medicine. To my good friend and colleague Charles O'Dean; thank you so much for your invaluable input into all my business projects, your sincerity, your sound advice and judgement in professional matters and simply 'telling like it is' – thank you. To Cass Gilroy, Editor of the African Echo; thank you for giving me the first real opportunity for publishing my articles – I have never forgotten your kindness nor your help in my foray into publishing as a novice writer. To my friend and colleague Dr. Clyde Wilson, Consultant Microbiologist at the King Edward Memorial Hospital in Bermuda; thank you so very much for all your help, support and immeasurable generosity. To Cyrus King from whom I learnt so much about natural remedies and the importance of nutrition – thank you. To Dr. Jayne Tullett, Chair of Endometriosis SHE Trust whose dedication, passion and drive to improve the lives of sufferers of endometriosis is truly commendable – it is a real pleasure to work with you. Also, a special thank you to Diane Carlton, former Chair of the Trust for the many professional collaborations.

I thank my colleagues David Potterton, Alex Laird, Prof. Jonathan Brostoff, Professor Emeritus at Kings College London, Claire McDonald at The Times, Dr. Celia Bell, Head of Department of Natural Sciences at Middlesex University, Dr. Kofi Busia, Technical Director at the West African Health Organisation (WAHO) and Dr. Michael Michaelides, Scientific Director at the Cyprus Sport Research Center.

A special thank you to my wonderful friends who have kept me sane and supported through good times and difficult moments: Farzana Anverkhan, Geneviève Robinson, Gina Yiannis, Sarah Browne, Wellington Sandiford, Michaela Becker, Ange Burrett, Caroline Abel, Linda Moran and Gemma Rattery.

CONTENTS

FOREWORD

I watched my mother suffer throughout her life from the effects of drugs prescribed and given to her. Side effects were dealt with by more drugs, producing more side effects. Just before she died, she was a part of a class action taken against a very well known drug company. They settled, but she passed on before she could reap any small benefit, apart from peace of mind. I don't bring this up as a swingeing attack on modern western medical practices - there is a place for allopathic medicine, of course. I bring it up because it broke my heart to see her suffer and it was a catalyst for my journey into Alternative remedies and Holistic Health. It was too late for my mother, but I became determined to be well and stay well. I wanted to know everything I could about supplements, herbal remedies, alternative practices, lifestyle management, nutrition, meditation and so on. It became a fascination.

We humans are miracles!

Just as, as an actress, I build a picture of the character I'm playing, piece by piece, putting her together from the text, research and of course my imagination, so I began to build a picture of how we work on an holistic level. And the more I learnt about how we work (and I don't know half of it), the more excited I became. We exist on so many levels: quantum, atomic, cellular, the whole organ, and of course the whole person. And that's before you consider the subtle energy fields we create, within and without. Nature has created a masterpiece and each masterpiece is unique. This is terribly important to understand, because Western medicine deals with universal symptoms or emergencies and not with individuals. The Holistic approach is for the individual and works with Nature instead of, as sometimes happens, against it.

So, when Yaso Shan, a Herbal Medicine consultant, author and practitioner of repute, with a serious scientific background contacted me about the book that she had written and asked if I would pen a foreword, I agreed with pleasure. At last – a book that was comprehensive enough to learn from, but not so full of jargon that the enthusiastic layman (me!) was put off. At the present time, questions are being asked both publicly and privately about herbal remedies, homeopathy, vitamin supplements and alternative practices generally. It is therefore very comforting to have a book that answers some of these questions with clarity and knowledge.

This book serves as evidence of the importance of medicinal plants in the treatment of patients and as a valid acknowledgement of the genuinely alternative ways to address healthcare. Yaso Shan delivers her verdicts with a sensitive appreciation for natural forms of medicine whilst acknowledging the medical and technological advancements within conventional healthcare. I recommend this book to anyone who wishes to gain an appreciation of the potential benefits of Western Herbal Medicine, to anyone who wants a better understanding of the therapeutic value of plants or quite simply, to anyone who seeks to learn something about effective, natural and alternative approaches to healthcare.

Jenny Seagrove

INTRODUCTION

An increasing number of people are becoming aware of health issues that affect them. As individuals take responsibility for their own health and being more proactive in ensuring their optimum well-being, there is a growing demand for products and services to reflect this trend. An example of this can be seen by the numerous health campaigns instigated by national and local organisations in addition to independent health agencies and charities. The proliferation of private health and fitness clubs is another example of the general level of interest shown and the responsibility taken by the public regarding their health and well being.

Equally of course, there have been recent controversies such as those surrounding the long-term health risks of GM foods, the concerns raised over the use of anabolic-type hormones, antibiotics and other potent chemicals in food preparation techniques. This is particularly the case for meat, poultry and fish, which may, to some extent account for the substantial market growth for organic produce. However, the cost implications of purchasing organic foods exclusively remain a huge consideration for the average household. The popular consensus is that given the choice, most people would prefer to purchase organic produce and primarily for health reasons than for any other. Similarly, other medical issues that have been highlighted in the media in recent times such as the concerns over the MMR vaccine, the health risks of certain vitamin and mineral supplements, the associated health risks of HRT, have all inadvertently favoured natural alternatives to preventing and treating illness in addition to the strategies adopted for optimising health and well-being.

Paradoxically, the growth in the health supplements market appears to contradict any concerns that the public may possibly have over supposed health risks with certain specified vitamin and mineral supplementation. Campaigners for consumer choice argue that the public retain the right to make well-informed decision regarding their health as well as the right to choose whatever is safe and effective. Additionally, responsible and objective reporting of controversial health issues is equally warranted so as not to unnecessarily alarm the public, through hidden agendas of large corporations, pharmaceutical companies and government policies. Fortunately, in a society where impartial and substantial information on health matters is readily available, especially now with internet service provision in most homes across the country, an increasing level of accountability and an increased access to information, individuals can realistically make well-informed choices regarding what is best for their own health and well being.

The health patterns in our society have also changed over the years and people are living longer. Current disease prevalence patterns reveal a recurrence of illnesses previously eradicated such as TB all show worrying signs of increase (especially in the UK). Equally worrying is the frequency of new strains of infectious organisms or 'superbugs' that are quite resistant to routine conventional treatment. It is perhaps one area where natural remedies such as herbal medicine may highlight their therapeutic potential in optimising health through increasing immune function in a climate where over-prescription of antibiotics has rendered the body rather incapable of resisting infection naturally. It becomes more pronounced in a hospital healthcare setting where the spread of such virulent superbugs that have become resistant to some of the more standard broad-spectrum antibiotics commonly prescribed for hospital acquired infections (eg. MRSA; (methicillin-resistant *Staphyloccus aureus*), *Clostridum difficile* (or *C.difficile* for short). Outbreaks of other infections such as *E.Coli* have also been a problem. Hospital-acquired illnesses are an acute problem and a serious cause for concern within primary health care. The problem may well be reflective of our reduced immune function and hence an increased susceptibility to disease; we no longer place our systems under important, necessary, and regular immunological challenges particular when our immediate domestic environment and lifestyles are too 'sterile'. This is the view argued by some of the leading medical immunologists and appears to be acknowledged and highly respected amongst other medical specialists too.

Technological advances in the 21st Century, particularly in the biomedical sciences, such as a stem cell therapy, gene cloning and gene therapy, have revolutionised medicine. Moreover, the applications of such techniques have transformed the quality of life of patients in respect of treating certain illnesses and diseases for which there was previously no effective treatment, alternatives or cure. Highly controversial in some instances (eg. hybrid embryo research) such techniques however, have profoundly altered the lives of many individuals for the better. The research potential in these new areas of medical science will continue to persist as long as illness and disease exists.

Notwithstanding the benefits of new medical technologies and as much as one may marvel at the pace of advancement in medical research and application, it is often the case that such developments and innovations directly conflict with public opinion and demand. Concerns over these issues seem to impact on the fundamental concept of what is considered healthy. As more and more people question conventional medical practices, particularly the indiscriminate prescription of drugs, public dissatisfaction in this practice has been paralleled by growing popularity in Complementary and Alternative Therapies. Many people are increasingly disenchanted with modern drug therapy and are becoming more open to traditional methods of treatment that is in keeping with nature, both in its design, effectiveness and principles. Many have also realised that science and conventional medicine does not have all the answers to all of the modern health problems and want to address the acute absence of spiritual health and well-being that exists in our societies which is directly linked to many of these health problems, particularly within mental health.

Moreover, some people are frustrated and disillusioned at the general level of medical service preferring to pay for the privilege of a lengthy discussion into their specific health problem with a diagnosis and treatment that is carried out within a holistic context. In spite of these differences however, medical science does have much to offer and in some cases, continues to provide the best and most effective treatment choice for the patient. Its role and purpose in these instances must be given due credit and respect.

Despite best intentions, there are many of us who are constrained by the modern lifestyle culture and it becomes extremely impractical, almost impossible to follow a relatively healthy lifestyle. The pressures of juggling work and family, particularly for working parents, means that the long term effects are undoubtedly going to have its toll on health and well-being. Reassuringly, the 24-hour culture similar to that of the US appears to be fast-growing in Britain and employers are more open to suggestions of flexible working patterns. The leisure industries including public and private gyms, health clubs and fitness centres now have extended opening hours enabling many to achieve a practical and realistic approach to adopting healthier lifestyles. Opportunities to address individual and specific health needs have never been better in terms of choice, flexibility, cost and convenience.

Diseases of the 21st Century such as heart disease, stroke, late onset diabetes (type 2 diabetes), clinical obesity and certain cancers look set to rise. Worryingly, some of these diseases, which are more commonly associated with age and decline show alarming signs of increase among the younger population. In a culture that perpetuates 'quick fixes' it is often tempting to address common health problems within our society with radical regimes. A classic case in point would be the previously popular Atkins Diet, which has divided medical opinion and has concerned many nutritionists, and alternative medical practitioners such as herbalists.

It is perhaps important to note that the Atkins Diet, when viewed in its entirety was intended to address the serious issue of Syndrome X, a clinical presentation which is characterised by chronic obesity, raised glucose levels (a form of type 2 diabetes) and other associated symptoms with potential health risks. It also proved to be effective at addressing the widespread problem of chronic obesity in America as a consequence of Western dietary practices and poor nutritional habits through excessive consumption of convenience foods. In the short term, it aimed to limit the potential life-threatening complications that result from excessive weight. Despite the risks of this diet, such as kidney failure and the possibility of cancer, it does provide a short-term, yet effective remedy to the altered metabolism that has resulted due to a prolonged exposure to poor dietary habits. However, only one aspect of the Atkins Diet was ever adopted and marketed on a wide scale therefore its full potential and its long-term benefits never materialised.

In raising important fundamentals on good nutritional practices and in encouraging better eating habits, particularly in the young, this book aims to better educate the public on such matters. In placing emphasis on making better choices regarding basic nutrition, perhaps the demand for such potentially risky 'quick fixes', though effective when administered and practiced correctly, would not be embraced with such fervour as it has been of late. Nor would it be that widespread especially amongst those who would benefit more from 'sensible' eating, balanced with moderate aerobic exercise. In advocating healthier lifestyle choices, particularly at a younger age, it is hoped that such diseases of the 21st Century that present with alarming statistics of fatalities and medical concerns could be addressed much earlier within our society. This would certainly halt some of the more fad diets that appears to capture public attention *en masse* but tends to resemble very much the approach of 'closing the stable door once the horse has bolted'.

This book caters for the person who has concerns about their general state of health, fitness and well-being. It caters for those who share concerns with other like-minded individuals about the indiscriminate use of prescription drugs for a number of common ailments that can be treated and most certainly prevented through natural and alternative methods including diet and lifestyle changes. It caters for those who want to improve their overall health and nutritional status. It is also for those who want to follow a more natural regime in respect of diet and lifestyle, in order that they can cope better with the numerous demands of modern living. Essentially, the book proposes to inform on the fundamentals of Western herbal medicine; its principles and practices within a holistic context giving due regard to the pressures and health consequences of modern living. It aims to introduce some basic concepts of treating with herbal remedies using the examples of a few of the more popular herbs. It aims to make suggestions for addressing some key aspects to good health and optimising well-being, such as improving digestion and liver function, boosting immunity and resistance to infection, regulating sleep, improving mood and increasing energy levels. There are suggestions of how herbal remedies can be incorporated into daily routines and practices in addition to some essentials on good nutrition, one of the foundations of maintaining optimum health.

In short, this book is aimed at those, like myself who share mutual concerns about the increasingly unnatural way in which we live, in addition to the long-term health risks of many conventional drugs that are routinely prescribed for a number of common ailments. It also aims to inform the public on the many simple measures that can be taken in order to counterbalance the enormous stresses that we are faced with on a daily basis owing to the pressures of work, family and home. It aims to provide a better understanding of health and ill-health through education on the basic and essential workings of the human body.

The complex undertaking of addressing all aspects of health and illness is beyond the scope of this book and it does not propose to replace some fundamental aspects of conventional medicine, which in context has an important remit and serves a crucial role in patient care, treatment and management. However, the book does discuss the many benefits of healthy living, practical measures for adopting healthier lifestyles and the many pressures of modern living that give rise to the multitude of symptoms so commonly seen and which can be easily prevented. It does offer a herbal alternative to most common problems and how to improve nutrition and make simple lifestyle changes in order to prevent and improve general health & well-being and ultimately improve quality of life.

Herbal Medicine is however, an Alternative form of medicine and hence should not be regarded in conjunction with conventional medicines as a complement to drug therapy. However, in some instances and under proper medical supervision, herbal medicine can serve as adjunct therapy to some chronic conditions, such as arthritis, hypertension or diabetes. I believe that there is a role for every kind of practitioner, be it conventional or alternative. In the current policy of improving services within the NHS there has come a time for seriously considering the role of the Medical Herbalist within the primary healthcare setting, particularly when through appropriate management and education, preventing illness and disease is one of the areas when the absolute effectiveness of Herbal Medicine can be viewed at its best. This can ultimately realise significant cost savings for the NHS through improving health & well-being, preventing illness and treating common problems with effective herbal medicines rather than prescribing strong and expensive drug treatments, or worse still, surgery.

It is my opinion that the discerning public are poorly informed about the therapeutic effectiveness, impact, usefulness and application of herbal remedies in the context of illness, both in its prevention and in treatment. This is one of the primary reasons for writing this book.

In placing the role of herbal medicine in relation to human form and function, I hope to enable individuals to better understand the basic workings of the body in respect of resistance to infection and improving major functions that are critical to preventing illness. It is envisaged that this, in time, will make clear how herbal medicine can enhance the natural healing process that exists as inherent mechanisms within our systems. In reviewing the biological fundamentals that govern health, well-being, illness and disease, and in advocating natural approaches to optimising health, the importance of herbal medicines can be easily identified.

Finally, it is intended that an exploration of the health trends and behavioural patterns in our society that directly impact on health and well-being can make clear the role of the medical herbalist in identifying many of the underlying causes of common physical problems. This is particularly the case when diagnosis is conducted within a holistic framework; very much in public favour when frequently, symptoms are mere manifestations of stress-related issues pertaining to the pressures of modern lifestyle and practices. All such factors will be closely examined in this book.

CHAPTER 1 – HEALTH & ILL-HEALTH

(i)   The Co-ordinated Body *(by Dr. Catherine Whitlock)*
(ii)   Understanding Illness *(by Dr. Catherine Whitlock)*
(iii)   Resistance to disease *(by Dr. Catherine Whitlock)*
(iv)   Modern lifestyle and disease/Symptoms of modern living (importance of sleep, mental health & wellbeing, mind-body link or PNI)

(i) The Co-ordinated Body

The human body is one of the most remarkable natural machines witnessed in the animal kingdom. Some of its inner workings are still a mystery, but scientists and clinicians are continually revealing information that helps us understand how diseases arise. In its simplest terms, the body operates on a structural (anatomical) level and on a functional (physiological level). Thus, the body becomes increasingly complex.

Chemicals → Cells → Tissues → Organs → Systems → Functioning Organism

One of the most important features of the human body is its ability to coordinate the multitude of systems contained within it. Cooperation between these is vital to a healthy body.

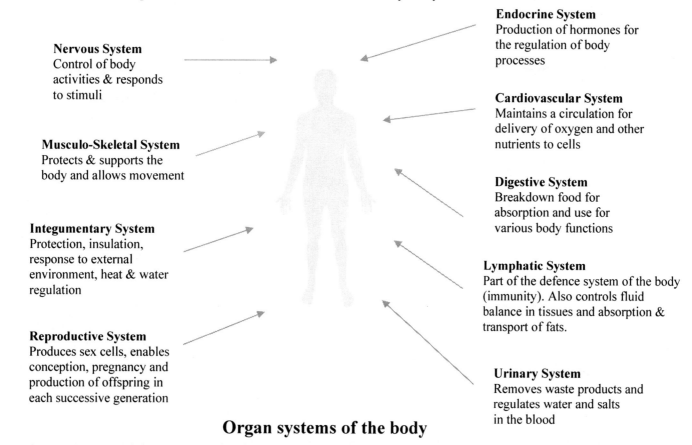

Nervous System
Control of body activities & responds to stimuli

Musculo-Skeletal System
Protects & supports the body and allows movement

Integumentary System
Protection, insulation, response to external environment, heat & water regulation

Reproductive System
Produces sex cells, enables conception, pregnancy and production of offspring in each successive generation

Endocrine System
Production of hormones for the regulation of body processes

Cardiovascular System
Maintains a circulation for delivery of oxygen and other nutrients to cells

Digestive System
Breakdown food for absorption and use for various body functions

Lymphatic System
Part of the defence system of the body (immunity). Also controls fluid balance in tissues and absorption & transport of fats.

Urinary System
Removes waste products and regulates water and salts in the blood

Organ systems of the body

Although these can be classified into different systems there is some overlap. For example, the ovaries form part of the endocrine and female reproductive systems. Each system interacts with others to ensure a healthy body. So, the endocrine glands release hormones directly into the cardiovascular system or bloodstream where they are transported directly to organs and tissues throughout the body. These hormones regulate metabolism, growth and sexual development. The endocrine and nervous systems work in tandem with each other to maintain effective communication of many of the body's processes, although they work at quite different speeds. Nerve signals (referred to as impulses) travel from the control centre, the brain, along the nerves of the nervous system at up to 250 miles per hour, while the endocrine system may take hours to respond with hormone production and the immune system days or even weeks to mount an appropriate response to an infection.

The lymphatic and cardiovascular systems are another example of closely related systems, joined by capillaries. 'Lymph' is a milky body fluid that contains both the cells of the immune system and proteins and fats. Lymph seeps outside the blood vessels into the spaces of body tissues and is stored in the lymphatic system to flow back into the bloodstream. The lymphatic system is important, not only to the immune system, because it drains excess fluids and protein so that tissues do not swell up.

Synergy is the key to optimum functioning of all these systems and the maintenance of health and well-being requires a careful balance or homeostasis. The holistic approach to diagnosis and treatment aims to examine the root cause of ill health by examining the levels of function and the context in which the person has fallen ill.

(ii) Understanding illness

Illness can be due to a number of factors and causative agents. For most people, the cause of illness is usually due to an infective agent. However, for this agent to cause illness requires a number of factors:

1. how powerful (or virulent) the infectious agent is (eg, bacteria, virus, fungus etc..)
2. the body's natural resistance to infection (natural immunity)
3. complication or secondary infections (following the primary infection or illness) which may be more serious or debilitating than the initial illness
4. the body's ability to fight the infection (immune defences)
5. the environment for recovery and aftercare

When one or more systems are thrown off balance, illness or disease can occur. A number of factors can cause disease, but the end result is a state in which the body's functions are disturbed.

Classifying individual diseases can be difficult but the following influences need to be considered when we consider why and how a disease develops and whether we can control this:

- Our **genetic** inheritance plays a big part in our susceptibility to whether we are likely to develop a disease or indeed how our bodies respond once a disease occurs. Some have a strong genetic component where a disease is caused directly by inheriting a gene from one or both parents e.g. sickle cell anaemia, cystic fibrosis, muscular dystrophy or haemophilia. Many diseases do not have such an obvious genetic linkage, but their dominance in some families, compared to others, suggests there is a strong genetic component. e.g. high blood pressure, certain cancers, asthma, multiple sclerosis, schizophrenia and Alzheimer's disease.

  Similarly, some conditions have a sex linkage so that only one sex gets the disease. For example with haemophilia, females acts as carriers for the gene and males inherit the condition. In the cases of diseases like rheumatoid arthritis, females are more likely to develop it.

- **Congenital** disorders arise after chromosomal abnormality (in the genetic make up), abnormal development in the womb, or by an inherited genetic abnormality, but always results in a child being born with the condition. Examples of these are Down's syndrome, spina bifida and cystic fibrosis respectively.

- **Degenerative** disorders occur as our bodies age and there is a progressive deterioration of a tissue or organ. Osteoarthritis, osteoporosis, Alzheimer's and Parkinson's disease are all directly related to this ageing process.

- **Environmental** triggers are instrumental in the development of many diseases. Industrial pollutants can be associated with disease development, asbestos exposure and the chronic lung disease asbestosis being a good example. But, there are more everyday examples where environmental pollution e.g. the widespread use of agricultural pesticides has been related to the increase in asthma and bronchitis. Similarly, lung cancer is predominantly associated with smoking. In considering the environment, our diets play a significant role in the development of a number of diseases. These range from deficiencies in our diets that can be responsible for conditions such as anaemia and a weakened immune response through to the numerous problems associated with high fat, highly processed western diets and obesity – heart disease, type 2 diabetes and cancer.

- **Metabolic** disorders are often related to diet, in particular in the strong link between obesity and the development of type 2 diabetes. The use of the term 'metabolic' describes any condition that is caused by an abnormality in the conversion or metabolism of one set of substances in the body to an end product. It can be congenital due to an inherited enzyme abnormality or acquired due to disease of an endocrine organ, such as the pancreas in type 2 diabetes. Phenylketonuria (PKU) is an inherited metabolic disorder which prevents the normal breakdown of protein foods. Unless treated by dietary restrictions, this results in a fatal build up of an amino acid (the building block of proteins) in the brain and babies are now routinely tested at birth for this disorder.

■ **Infectious** diseases are caused by entry of a pathogen (infectious agent) or foreign organism/invader into the body. There are four main groups of infectious agents: viruses, bacteria, parasites and fungi. Examples of common or well known infectious diseases are given in the table below.

Characteristics of some common, or well known, infectious diseases

Pathogen		Disease	Route of infection	Symptoms
Type	Name			
Bacteria.	*Salmonella typhii*	Food poisoning	Food and water	Vomiting/Diarrhoea
	Chlamydia trachomatis	Chlamydia infection	Sexually transmitted	Often symptomless, but may result in mild irritation and pain and discharge in both sexes. Can cause pelvic inflammatory disease and result in blocked fallopian tubes and hence infertility.
	Staphlococcus aureus	Impetigo	Skin contact	Red itchy patches turning to crusty yellow skin lesions
Virus	*Influenza virus type A, B or C.*	Flu	Airborne water droplets	Fever, muscle pain, fatigue, headache and other cold-like symptoms.
	Herpes simplex I or *Herpes simplex II*	Mouth or genital cold sores.	Mouth or genital contact	Tingling painful sores or lesions occur after the primary infection and also every time the virus, which lies dormant in the skin, is triggered to replicate.

	Varicella zoster	Chicken pox. Shingles	Contact with infected person. Initial infection results in chicken pox. Life long immunity to chicken pox recurrence, but virus persists in nerve endings and can reactivate as shingles.	Chicken pox - Itchy red spots that crust over as the disease progresses. Shingles – painful rash often localised on the trunk.
Fungus	*Tinea pedis*	Athelete's foot	Picked up in warm damp areas, such as swimming pool changing rooms.	Itchy, white, flaky rash in moist areas eg. between the toes
	Candida albicans	Thrush	Direct contact esp. during sexual contact (genital thrush) or breastfeeding (oral thrush in infants)	Genital thrush, particularly vaginal thrush in women involves itching, and a white discharge. Oral thrush presents as white patches in the mouth
Parasite	Threadworm *Enterobious vermicularis*	Gut infection	Oral route as worm eggs under the finger nails are transferred into the gut to complete the life cycle	Itchy anus often at night as adult emerges to lay eggs
	Plasmodium - 4 types	Malaria	Complex life cycle with mosquito and human as the 2 hosts. Parasite passes between the	Several forms of disease, but recurrent fevers and flu-like symptoms common.

			hosts, as the saliva of a biting mosquito is transferred into the human bloodstream.	*Plasmodium falciparum* form of the disease infects the brain and can be fatal.

It is obvious that in considering why and how diseases develop there are many components. Cancer is often multifactorial in origin, that is, a number of different factors may cause or contribute to the disease. Many cancers have a strong genetic component, with predisposition to breast cancer and bowel cancer for example running in families. Others are linked to environmental exposure to mutagens such a lung cancer and smoking, and diet and bowel cancer. Heart disease is another example where diet, genetic inheritance and smoking for example are all risk factors.

In many diseases, particularly those caused by infections, the immune system plays a part in controlling the outcome and an understanding of how this works is vital to our treatment of those conditions.

(iii) Resistance to disease

The function of the immune system is to protect the body from damage caused by invading organisms – bacteria, viruses, fungi and parasites. This defensive function is performed by white blood cells and a number of accessory cells, which are distributed throughout the body, but are found particularly in lymphoid organs, including the bone marrow, thymus, spleen and lymph nodes. Large accumulations of these cells are also found at sites where pathogens enter the body, such as the mucosa of the gut or lung. Cells migrate between these tissues via the blood stream and lymphatic system. As they do so they interact with each other to generate coordinated immune responses aimed at eliminating pathogens or minimising the damage they cause.

The principal at the heart of the immune system is its ability to distinguish self from non-self. This is an ancient property of organisms and some sort of primitive immune response can be traced back in evolution to the earliest simple organisms like sponges. These contain immune cells that engulf and kill bacteria.

Each of us is born with a natural or innate immunity, the earliest evolutionary form of immunity. The cells and molecules that make up this initial response to a pathogen are neither specific to that organism nor improved by repeated encounters with the same agent. This is in contrast to adaptive or acquired immunity, which is specific for that particular pathogen and to the individual who generated it and is marked by an enhanced response on re-exposure. We are born with natural immunity, but adaptive immunity occurs over time as we are exposed to pathogens. A newborn baby gets a helping hand in this process if a mother breastfeeds.

So, the important features of the adaptive immune response are memory and specificity. In practise there is considerable overlap between the two arms of the immune response, but the principal of vaccination relies heavily on the adaptive immune response. Vaccinations contain a form of the pathogen that will not cause the disease, but does stimulate the immune cells; they are primed to react more quickly and to a greater degree when they encounter that pathogen in the future, thus fending off the illness.

The immune system consists of a multitude of molecules and cells that operate in a network, with many feedback and control mechanisms in place. This coordinated system is akin to solid organs like the kidney or a liver, but immune cells are unique in their ability to traffic or travel around the body. This is central to their patrolling, vigilant nature and has important implications for the development of subsequent, rapid and efficient immune responses. If a white blood cell encounters the flu virus in the lungs, for example, it will develop certain properties, a form of molecular memory that will allow that cell to immediately home back to the lung if it encounters that infection again.

The respiratory tract is one of the most common ways infections can enter the body. Airborne infections such as the cold and influenza virus are transmitted in water droplets contained in a person's sneeze or on infected hands. But there are other systems that infectious organisms can gain entry into, such as the digestive system and the reproductive systems, where for example Salmonella food poisoning and sexually transmitted diseases such as HIV AIDS can strike respectively. One of the many functions of the skin, and the mucous membranes such as those in the mouth, is to act as a barrier against infection. Bites, scratches, or puncture wounds that break the skin can increase the risk of infection, or be a direct route of entry such as the malaria parasite in the saliva of a biting mosquito.

As pathogens/infectious organisms can gain entry into the body in so many places, the body has to be prepared and the lymphatic system and its associated lymphoid tissue are vital to the functioning of a healthy immune system. The lymphoid organs are comprised of the bone marrow and thymus where the immune cells first develop and then the spleen and lymph nodes, where these cells are programmed to deal with an infection. The lymph nodes are dotted all over the body (see diagram below) as more than 100 tiny oval structures, packed full of white blood cells.

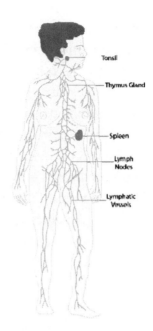

Tonsil

Thymus Gland

Spleen

Lymph
Nodes

Lymphatic
Vessels

The lymphatic system

These cells are numerous in their type and function, but three types are worthy of mention here: dendritic cells, T and B lymphocytes. The immune system responds to invading pathogens in a number of ways to try and rid the body of the infection. But we can use an example to illustrate the types of processes that take place. If a cut in the skin gets infected with bacteria, the dendritic cell found just below the skin's surface will engulf that bacteria, travel to the lymph node that drains that site and there it will present the bacteria in a form that can be recognised by T lymphocytes. These then 'help' B lymphocytes to make antibody to deal with the infections. If the initial infection is with a virus, T cells that kill the virally infected cell will be activated by the dendritic cell, and so on. The immune system has a whole armoury of mechanisms at its disposal.

The immune system takes time to mount the immune response and in that incubation period (which varies from hours to weeks depending on the pathogen), there may not be any symptoms but a patient may be highly infective. This is particularly true in the case of viruses as they replicate in the cells of the body, often shedding large quantities of virus e.g. the cold virus emerges in water droplets every time someone sneezes. How effective the treatments are, conventional or alternative, will partly depend on what stage the infection is caught. There's no doubt that most treatments are at their most effective just before or just after the person is infected, where levels of the pathogen are low in the body.

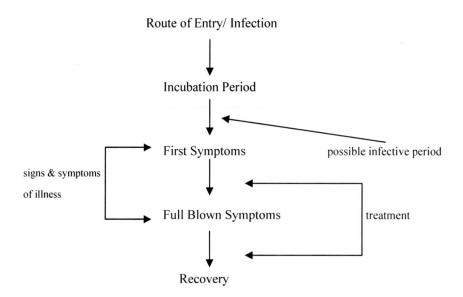

Simple schematic diagram showing the infection process and the pattern of disease

This is where herbal medicine may have a part to play in boosting the natural immune defences. Equally there are a number of important immune boosters contained in herbal preparations that combat infections directly, through their anti-microbial or anti-viral activity, helping to destroy and aid the removal of pathogens.

In dealing with infectious diseases, the immune system is behaving as our friend. But there are circumstances where the immune system works against us and as such it becomes our foe. This is what occurs when autoimmune diseases such as rheumatoid arthritis, systemic lupus erythematosus (SLE), multiple sclerosis (MS) and the autoimmune form of diabetes (type 1 diabetes) develop. There may be a genetic component and/or an infection that triggers their development, but what lies at the heart of the autoimmune disease process is the body attacking itself. The body produces antibodies or immune cells that react against the body's own components. There is a fundamental breakdown in that key feature of the immune system, to distinguish self from non-self.

Allergies can also be seen as a way in which the immune system acts against us. An allergic response occurs when the immune system reacts to a substance that is basically harmless or does not cause an immune response in everybody. Common allergens are often air borne such as pollen. In susceptible individuals, on encounter with these allergens, the immune system goes into overdrive producing antibodies and soluble molecules such as histamines. It is these histamines that are responsible for the sneezing, itchy eyes and sore throat that characterises many a summer for hay fever sufferers. Other allergens are contained within food products e.g. nuts, and in the most severely infected individuals, anaphylaxis can take place. This reaction is at the extreme end of the allergic spectrum and adrenaline injections are needed to control the symptoms of difficulty in breathing or swallowing and the drop in blood pressure that can often take place.

The prevalence of allergies is rising in the Western world. A number of scientists believe that the so-called hygiene hypothesis may explain this. As we have seen, the immune system exercises itself eliminating harmful pathogens but our increasingly clean lives means that we are not stimulating the immune system appropriately. The hygiene hypothesis proposes that exposure to allergen early in life reduces the risk of developing allergies by boosting immune system activity. A study that backs this up is that of children on German farms who regularly encountered a range of potential pathogens in the farmyard and who were found to have a significantly lower incidence of allergies such as hay fever.

Balance in the types of immune cells activated is crucial to understanding these ideas. When we encounter infectious diseases and when autoimmune diseases occur, a type of helper T lymphocyte is activated called the Th1 cell. Conversely, allergies are associated with a Th2 response. When the hygiene hypothesis was first proposed in the 1980s, it did not explain the rise in incidence of autoimmune diseases. The alternative explanation is that the developing immune system must receive stimuli (from infections) in order to prime a third type of T cell, described recently as the regulatory T cell. If this cell is not adequately stimulated, the body will be more susceptible to both autoimmune diseases and allergies, because neither the Th1 or Th2 responses are sufficiently repressed by this regulatory T cell.

There are of course some obvious exceptions to this theory in the form of the problems in hospitals of bacteria that are resistant to antibiotics, such as methicillin resistant *Staphylococcus aureus* (MRSA), reminding us that we need to strike a balance. Cleanliness is imperative in a hospital environment, when illness is prevalent and the immune system of patients may be suppressed and vulnerable to attack.

Balancing the stimulation of the immune response is very important. In the developing world, allergies and autoimmune diseases are rarer than in developed countries. The immune system is too busy fighting off dangerous pathogens, those organisms that cause malaria, AIDS, tuberculosis, schistosomiasis and leishmaniasis. The trade off here is that many of these diseases can and often are fatal.

Scientists are increasingly realising that the immune system, like every system in the body, does not act in isolation. Examples abound of clear links between mind and body at a molecular level. Immune molecules called cytokines can initiate brain actions. There are direct contacts between nerve fibres and lymphoid organs. And scientists have shown that a chemical signal which normally allows nerve cells to communicate with each other (to alter sleep cycles) can also redirect actions of the immune system. Similarly, the endocrine system works closely with the immune system so that chemicals that disrupt the endocrine system may also decrease resistance to disease. These examples all serve to remind us that focusing on our lifestyle provides an opportunity to influence our immune responses for the better. Our immune responses are strongly influenced by our genetic inheritance, our previous exposure to a pathogen, and how virulent or powerful that particular pathogen is. But, there are other factors that affect their efficiency – diet, stress, sleep (or lack of it), exercise and increasing age. A cold virus will infect a body when it is exposed to it, regardless of all these factors, but how the body deals with it, is related to all of them.

(iv) Modern Lifestyle and Disease/ Symptoms of Modern Living

Over the past few years, our lifestyles have become increasingly busy, with many of us juggling home and work within the demands of a family, financial commitments and friends. Priority for health is probably the last thing on most people's minds and the concept of good nutrition and maintaining a work-life balance is often overlooked amidst these pressures and the 'daily grind'.

Quite often I see patients exhibiting the typical pattern of what I describe as 'symptoms of modern living'. These symptoms are often numerous and quite insidious in nature, that is, it takes some time for the person to notice them and when they do, it has manifested after a number of years. Many of us can probably relate to the effects of poor sleep and mood disorders, particularly depression which is currently a big problem in modern, western society. Symptoms such as frequent headaches, skin rashes, anxiety, panic attacks and digestive problems are becoming increasingly common. Many of these will be discussed later in the book.

In addressing the health conditions within a holistic context it is important to examine our diet, our lifestyle, stress, sleep and the notion of a mind-body link. Our mental well-being is inextricably linked to our physical state (and *vice versa*) and modern science has made it possible for us to better understand the influences of factors such as stress on our physical and mental well-being.

The table below lists some common examples of symptoms people frequently suffer from but may not have attributed them to the way they live or describe any aspect of their life being possible causal factors.

Symptom	Possible cause(s) linked to a modern lifestyle	Comment
Headache	Stress, computer glare	Long hours on the computer causes eye strain and combined with work stress is a guarantee for an instant headache
Acne & other skin complaints eg. eczema	Stress, diet, hormonal imbalance	Stress plays havoc on hormone production and balance. This can lead to a variety of skin disorders, particularly acne which has an established hormonal link
Digestive symptoms (various) eg. heartburn,	Stress, diet, lifestyle	The classic picture of stress & anxiety coupled with a poor diet over a period of time leading to a host of digestive

		symptoms (can be acute or chronic)
Mood disorders eg. depression, irritability, aggression	Stress, lifestyle, food	Many causes & predisposing factors. Also consider the 'junk food junkie' which can explore the link between food & behaviour
Anxiety	Stress, depression, debt	Personality type has some bearing on those affected by everyday stressors but in other cases, there are outside factors and stress management and herbal anxiolytics can help a great deal in coping
Insomnia & other sleep disorders	Stress, anxiety, lifestyle	Can lead to irritability, fatigue & depression
Irritable bowel syndrome (IBS)	Diet, lifestyle, stress	Personality type & stress management must be considered as part of the treatment
Premenstrual Syndrome (PMS)	Stress, diet	Hormonal imbalances can be brought on through poor diet and stress
Fatigue	Long working hours, travel stress	A host of causes but simple fatigue or extreme tiredness through overwork and travel can deplete the body's energy reserves. Proper rest & recuperation is essential in repair, regeneration and rejuvenation of vital body functions

It is unsurprising to see that stress appears to be a predominant feature in all of the common symptoms listed above. Almost all of us are affected by stress in our daily lives and most adopt practical measures to cope with the effects of stress. Learning to manage stress and the daily stressors we face is the only way to achieve an adequate sense of well-being, both physically and mentally. The importance of the mind-body link cannot be sufficiently emphasised. Recent advances in the field of psychoneuroimmunology (PNI) has elucidated much in the manner in which the mind and body are linked and the intricate interrelationship between the two. The holistic philosophy would very much subscribe to this notion and many would say this is common sense. However, to have our suspicions and long-held beliefs confirmed by scientific evidence reinforces opinion and can profoundly influence the manner in which disease and illness is viewed and treated.

The study and understanding of pychoneuroimmunology (PNI) has resulted in innovative ideas and concepts to emerge regarding the biological basis of disease. The mind-body link has been shown to be influential in a number of disorders with physical and psychological manifestations. Crucially, the reduced immune responses following nervous and hormonal activation significantly increase the risk of infection and disease. It has been demonstrated that our normal coping mechanisms and adaptation following exposure to stress is substantially altered or disrupted in disease states. Such disease states have important influences from the higher centres in the brain (the limbic system and the higher cortical centres). Many of the alternative and complementary therapy principles enable a truly integrated approach to diagnosis and treatment which is very much limited in the Western medical model. In this respect, cognitive behavioural therapy (CBT) is of clinical value especially in cases associated with problems of social or personal adjustment rather than of organic disease (ie. mental rather than physical origin). This is also relevant where established patterns of behaviour have overwhelming emotional triggers. The schematic diagram on page 22 illustrates the role of the limbic system, a specific part of the brain which dictates our emotional and physical responses to various stimuli. The diagram also highlights where CBT could help.

Exploration of the human self at all levels of being must give due recognition to the subtle energies or anatomy, in addition to the implicate order of matter that consolidates the mind, body and spirit, as one. PNI attempts to seek scientific reasoning behind energy medicine but it is probably the case that the latter is more complex than can be quantified or proven within accepted scientific criteria. A truly integrated approach to medical conditions (disorders) would consider the multidimensional aspects of a person (or the subtle anatomy) utilising scientific discovery to enhance therapeutic effectiveness within a holistic framework.

Stress, Conditioning and Immunity

Immunologists have suspected an association between stress and immune function for many years but it is only relatively recently (with the advances in scientific research and technology) that the biological basis of a link has been established. However, the nerve and hormonal pathways involved in the behavioural alteration of immune responses are not yet known. There are a number of theories on both conditioning and stress-induced effects which involve a range of important biological compounds such as adrenocortical steroids, opioids and catecholamines, amongst others. Indeed, all of these have been implicated in the mediation of some immunological effects observed under some experimental conditions.

Based on the complexity of the network of connections and regulatory feedback loops between the brain and immune system, these processes appear to involve both nervous and hormonal signals to the immune system. Signals to the immune system that are received by the nervous system provoke further adjustments in the nervous and hormonal systems. Repeated stress exposure can lead to habituation of a physiological response. However, this does not mean that the ability to react to a new stimulus has declined. Despite stress exerting direct effects on brain anatomy, determining whether such anatomical changes alters the subsequent response to stress needs to be established. Moreover, human studies reveal that a subject's early experiences with stress and degree of coping skills will influence the effect of either acute or chronic stress on immune function. Equally, further studies are needed to determine whether chronic stress is associated with a predisposition to disease that involves the immune system.

Conditioned responses as demonstrated in 1975 by two scientists working in the field of PNI research (Robert Ader & Nicholas Cohen) showed that it is possible to adapt behaviour in a conditioned manner following a particular stress. In respect of gut pathologies and using the 'taste-aversion conditioning model' in animals, they demonstrated that the conditioned response may explain the association of some of the bowel disorders to chronic stress exposure. Immune adaptation may alter normal gut function over time, making the body more susceptible to disease via alterations in immune-mediated responses. The question is in determining the predisposed state rather than the immune association which has previously been established.

Personality and Disease Risk

The concept of personality type and disease risk has been speculated for some time and generates much discussion within psychology, particularly when there is significant crossover with biosocial factors and early childhood events. The psychological focus of personality will not be discussed here but it is fair to say that through observational studies, strong correlations are in fact present between the following: repressed emotions and hopelessness in cancer, hostility and aggression in heart disease, higher prevalence of neurotic and introverted types in ulcerative colitis (UC) and alexithymia (the inability to talk about feelings due to a lack of emotional awareness) in Inflammatory Bowel Disease (IBD). Previous studies have lacked scientific rigour, primarily due to the time constraints involved in conducting research; most studies were carried out over a 10-40 year period. The main stumbling block is very much in repeating such experiments over the same timescale (a true acid test!). At present therefore, one can only surmise and note the obvious observational links that occur between personality type and disease risk. There may be a generic 'disease-prone personality' where imbalances in personality may function like diet predisposing the individual to a host of diseases.

Following appropriate stressors, the higher centres in the brain and associated nerve pathways are undoubtedly activated. The consequential immunomodulatory effects may be implicated in many gut disorders of unknown mechanism. With reference to cancer development and immunity, strong evidence links the influence of catecholamines (such as adrenaline) and glucocorticoids (such as cortisol) on the distribution and functional capacity of a particular type of immune cell called the Natural Killer (NK) cell. Stress in particular, was shown to suppress NK cell activity in all established stress studies. Additionally, stress was also shown to affect other factors that may facilitate tumour development and spread; such unknown characteristics of the host may determine whether factors other than NK cells play a role in initiating the spread of cancer (a long held suspicion is that it does). Similar studies add to a growing body of evidence that makes a unique contribution towards understanding the effects of stress on NK cell activity and its role in cancer.

Emotional Aspects in Gastroenterology

The focus here has been on gut pathologies because the disorders are so common and it is where the link between the mind and body is best illustrated. Emotion covers a substantial and significant area of psychology and by definition alone it encompasses both the mental and the physical. The limbic system and the hypothalamus in the brain are in essence the mediators of emotional expression and feelings, with the external expression of emotional content being represented by the 'affective' state. Repressed emotions (as previously mentioned in cancer risk) are in fact associated with psychosomatic disease; the most important in this context are anger, sense of dependency and fear.

Negative emotional states have been strongly implicated in illness and it is of significance in gut pathologies owing to the established mind-gut axis. The amygdala and hippocampus are important structures within the limbic system which provides a biological basis for some of the physical manifestations with overriding emotional associations. Of relevant discussion here is that the amygdala and hippocampus which can both be influenced by psychological intervention. CBT principles are based very much on this aspect of treatment. Though the memory of past events remains constant in the amygdala, the response to it (following appropriate triggers) can change over time. The part of the brain controlling voluntary behaviour is therefore crucial in overriding this. In altering the response manner to emotional triggers, CBT can influence the amygdala to discern the relevance of the stimuli (stress response) whenever evoking the same response (see schematic diagram below).

Alternative and Complementary Therapies in PNI

A clearer understanding of principal pathways in PNI has enabled the application of a variety of alternative and complementary therapies that operate either at the level of the mind, the neurendocrine (nerve signalling and hormonal) level or at the immune level. Such therapies may have indirect consequential effects or conversely, directly intervene key mechanistic PNI pathways. Concepts and approaches are essentially dependent on the fundamental principles of each therapy, and too broad to address within this book.

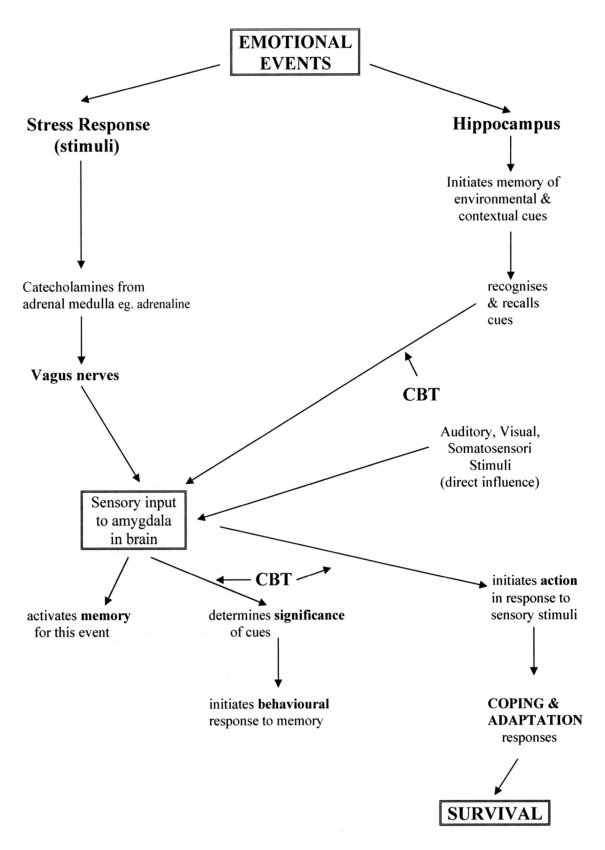

Schematic representation of the role of the brain's limbic system in emotional and physical responses in the normal physiological state

Exploration of mind-body pathways and the biological mechanisms that operate within PNI has provided fresh perspectives to current disorders within gastroenterology. A truly integrated approach will combine aspects of these together with fundamental concepts within the Western medical model in the diagnosis and treatment of such disorders. Equally, respecting the subtle energies at work in individual presentations of illness should give latitude to influences that fall outside the reductionist viewpoint. Purporting the mind-body-spirit concept with emotional and behavioural consequences draws comparables to traditional Eastern medical paradigms that appear to be embraced with fervour in the West.

Mere amelioration of physical manifestations (symptoms) is simply insufficient if true harmony between the physical body, the psychological (behaviour and emotion) and spiritual being (subtle anatomy) is to be considered in its entirety. Lack of empirical data on an interdependent interaction between all three aspects does not preclude its existence. Neither should the mind-body-spirit be regarded as an autonomous concept devoid of scientific reasoning or principle. In fact, disease is very much an imbalance of these 3 aspects of 'being'. Examining primitive behaviour patterns, basic instinctive reactions, gender bias and environment can all provide vital clues in the relative preponderance of current disease states. Deviation from our natural tendencies within the context of our 'civilised' societies and modern lifestyles should undoubtedly be a significant consideration in any clinical assessment.

The holistic management will thus account for these factors in addition to emphasising the unequivocal importance of the therapeutic relationship. This may require deep introspection on both sides that imbues a conducive environment for healthy, interactive dialogue, thus providing a safe and effective forum for healing at all levels of the human self.

Sleep

Modern lifestyle can also affect sleep, another very important aspect of our well-being. So many of us are not getting the right amount or quality of sleep. This is not surprising since the impact of stress and modern living can make it impossible to mentally 'switch off' until our bodies are physically exhausted. By that stage of course it may well be too late and the impact of sleep deprivation may have started to kick in. The symptoms of inadequate sleep can vary from irritability, mood swings and depression to recurrent colds, decline in mental alertness and acuity plus a host of other problems. The clinical picture will vary for each person depending on the susceptibility of their bodies to these symptoms and addressing these problems will require a close assessment of lifestyle, diet, the impact of stress and other factors such as the environment, relationships and personal circumstances.

The purpose of sleep

The physiological importance of sleep is essentially to restore, regenerate, rejuvenate and revitalise. It is also the time for growth and repair, a crucial aspect for optimum health. In higher animals such as humans, the nervous system is very advanced and requires considerable rest and restoration, particularly if the cells have been active throughout the day.

The Sleep Cycle

The sleep cycle is just that, a cycle of events. It alternates between stages of deep sleep and periods of arousal or wakefulness called REM or the rapid eye movement stage. REM is described as a state of wakefulness or a state of arousal because sleep is potentially dangerous for animals such as humans and this alternating pattern is crucial because it forms the basis of survival; prolonging the deep sleep stage can make the person go into a coma and ultimately death. The diagram below shows a simple representation of the cyclical events during the sleep cycle.

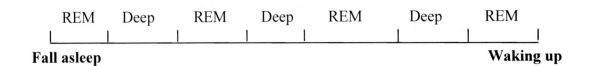

Schematic diagram of The Sleep Cycle highlighting the alternating and repeating pattern of deep sleep and REM which is characterized by rapid eye movements

Invariably, dreams occur during the periods of REM. The duration of the REM stages increases as the night progresses and it is common to wake up in the middle of a dream. People are able to remember their dreams more vividly when they happen at the latter REM stages rather than those earlier in the night. We only require about 2 stages of deep sleep and the longest of these happen at the early stages of sleep, more or less as soon as we fall asleep. Most of the rest, regeneration, repair and growth occur during these deep sleep stages On average, a healthy adult would need about 7-8 hours of sleep, children requiring more and the elderly requiring less.

Sleep is dependent on hormones and the control of nerve signaling. This means that it is regulated by hormones, particularly melatonin (which is secreted at night) and the nervous system (which is controlled and activated by the brain or higher centres).

The symptoms of sleep deprivation

The symptoms of a lack of adequate sleep, particularly the deep sleep can vary from mild or moderate to severe. Prolonged bouts of sleep disturbances or lack of sleep has a detrimental effect on the body, particularly in the long-term. It is important to address the root cause of any sleep abnormalities to prevent these symptoms and as the table below highlights, they can be numerous and can have a damaging effect on our well-being and function.

- Poor concentration and attention span
- Reduced mental alertness
- Reduced mental acuity
- Confusion
- Lack of energy
- Fatigue & exhaustion
- Emotional & psychological symptoms eg. depression, melancholia, anger, irritability
- Headache
- Reduced immune function & increased susceptibility to infection
- Visual disturbances
- Reduced memory
- Reduced problem-solving abilities
- Poor co-ordination & balance

Sleep pathologies

The main problem that people encounter with sleep is not getting enough of it! Some find it difficult to get to sleep but will sleep well thereafter. Others will wake up in the middle of the night and find it difficult to get back to sleep. This can leave them feeling unwell and un-refreshed the following morning. Some will drift in and out of sleep all night and again, this will also leave the sufferers feeling un-refreshed and groggy in the mornings.

Taking prescription sleeping tablets (eg. barbiturates and tranquilizers) provide little long-term solution especially in those with chronic sleep disorders. These drugs will suppress both deep sleep and REM phases of sleep which is one reason why people feel even more sleepy the next day. Examining the root causes of insomnia is essential if the problem is to be successfully tackled. Further aspects of sleep and the role of herbal sedatives and hypnotics will be discussed in the chapter 5, Health Essentials.

Mood

Sleep is inextricably linked to mood and as indicated earlier, a lack of sleep, particularly on a regularly basis will profoundly affect our outlook on life and general mood. The description of mood is somewhat subjective and some aspects of it are largely determined by personality, upbringing and life experiences. However, a sense of well-being is linked to a positive approach to things and many factors other than a lack of sleep will also influence mood. Some of these other factors have been listed below.

- Work pressures and unemployment
- Environment (home or work)
- Relationships (family, partner or friends)
- Poor diet

- Alcohol
- Lifestyle (eg. lack of exercise)
- Sexual problems

Mental health is a significant aspect of our well-being and optimum health. A healthy mind is just as important as our physical health.

Energy

The concept of energy is a complex one and its definition has many dimensions. In its metaphysical sense, it defined as the ability of any particulate matter to do work. Its property is such that it cannot be created nor destroyed, merely to change from one form to another. This describes the first law of conservation and something that forms the basis of all living things and matter.

Most of us have some understanding that in order for the human body to function effectively, then it must be fuelled by energy. Modern life can deplete vital energy resources through poor diet, stress, illness, our environment, lack of exercise and poor sleep. These are just a few of the many factors that govern our body's ability to do work and determine whether it is efficient or indeed effective in its many physiological functions. Having an abundance of energy is a goal that most of us share and we equate it to a kind of vitality that represents positive health.

However, modern living can make this impossible. This is why most of us feel lethargic, exhausted, and lack enthusiasm for life. To restore this 'lost' energy we need to take a long hard look at what is not working in our lives and to either discard it or to change it. Equally, it is important to examine all that is positive and good, and then find ways to embrace it, to enhance it or to improve it.

As explained earlier in the chapter, the mind has a profound influence over the body so examining all aspects of one's life must focus on the mental, physical, emotional, spiritual and psychological. A positive attitude to health can work miracles on our energy levels. In aiming to achieve this positive state of mind, we must attempt to do the following:

- Identify factors in our lives that deplete our energy resources
- Identify factors in our lives that cause negative stress
- Maximize our energy potential and sense of well-being
- Examine the way in which we view our bodies. We must learn to view our body not as a sum of different parts but as an integrated whole with a mind, body and spirit connection
- Learn to view the changes in our health status, fluctuating between positive and negative influences in the environment
- Be aware of warning signs that the body sends out. A lack of energy is a classic sign of many physiological disorders. Signs and symptoms are the body's way of communicating

to us that something is wrong. We cannot afford to ignore it as it is a guaranteed way to ask for trouble. Taking affirmative action at the critical time will avoid problems later on.

Some of the influences on our energy reserves:

Sleep – as explained earlier, poor sleep, particularly as lack of deep sleep deprives the body of its ability to repair and regenerate. This in turn, will impact on how the body can restore its energy reserves.

Diet – having an unhealthy diet, particularly one that is loaded with saturated fats and simple carbohydrates will not nourish the body or fuel the body sufficiently for work.

Mood – profoundly influences the energy levels in the body (and *vice versa*). Can be a very complex issue to address and getting the right professional help for some of the mental health disorders can sometimes be the only way forward

Environment – toxins, pollutants, chemicals, water and even medication can all lead to 'toxic overload'. This in turn will deplete our energy reserves and impact on our basic body functioning

Illness – medication can make us tired, as can illness itself

Lifestyle – the way we live has a powerful influence on our energy levels eg. excessive alcohol consumption, smoking, lack of exercise, inadequate sleep all have a detrimental effect on our energy and ultimately on our health in general

Stress – we all want to achieve the perfect 'work-life balance' and very few of us actually achieve it. The impact of stress cannot be sufficiently stated. The adverse effects of stress have a significant impact on our energy and ultimately our general health and well-being. Combating the negative effects of stress is part of the work of many holistic therapists in attempting to achieve the ultimate work-life balance and in examining the person in the context of their illness.

CHAPTER 2 – HOLISTIC HEALTH

(i)   Definition & philosophy of (Western) Herbal Medicine (synergy of active ingredients etc..)
(ii)   Treating the 'whole person' – a holistic approach to diagnosis and treatment
(iii)   A brief history of herbal medicine & cultural contexts of practice
(iv)   Prevention, cure and herbal medicine (helping the body to heal itself)

(i) Definition and philosophy of Western Herbal Medicine

Herbal Medicine is an ancient worldwide practice of using plants to prevent and cure disease. Records dating as far back as 2000BC suggest the use of healing plant remedies and some of the more traditional cultures in the world still practice herbal medicine as the main form of treatment in infection and disease. In more recent and scientific times, attempts have been made to recognise the true importance and value of medicinal plants; after all, two thirds of all conventional drugs are from plant origin. Analysing chemical constituents of medicinal plants and conducting experimental trials has led to a better understanding of their actions. From such studies, it becomes clear that it is the synergistic action of their active ingredients that plays a crucial role in explaining their effectiveness. That is to say, the sum of these active parts in the plant as a whole, has a greater therapeutic effect that any of the isolated active ingredients on their own.

Despite the fact that much of the medical and popular literature on herbal medicines is difficult to interpret, we should keep an open mind and accept that although a substance may lack evidence of effectiveness, it does not imply that it is ineffective. Neither does it mean that it cannot be useful in any medical condition or illness. A lack of *evidence* of effect is not the same as lack of effect and an unproven herb can nevertheless be beneficial for many patients and for many disorders. Although the overall evidence for many herbal medicines is often markedly deficient or of unacceptably poor quality, the efficacy and safety of an increasing number of potentially useful herbal products have been evaluated in well-designed clinical studies, including randomised controlled trials and systematic reviews.

Encouragingly, the trend for conducting large-scale trials is changing, particularly in the US where the National Center for Complementary and Alternative Medicine (NCCAM) at the National Institutes for Health (NIH) has dramatically increased their budget for research in recent years. The NCCAM now funds large-scale randomised controlled trials on:

St. John's Wort
Ginkgo
Echinacea
Saw palmetto

Botanical research is also being conducted on a host of other herbal supplements such as:

Soy
Red clover
Black cohosh
Ginger
Turmeric
Boswellia
Grape polyphenols
Green tea

The fundamental philosophy of Western herbal medicine is essentially one of promoting good health and treating illness through the use of medicinal plants, either in their whole form or as concentrates of their active ingredients. The healing process is carried out within a holistic context and utilises the principle of enabling the body to heal itself. So the focus can be on enhancing liver function, boosting circulation or improving immune responses, all of which are natural biological functions in the maintenance of good health and vitality.

Basic Principles & Practice of Western Herbal Medicine

Western cultures have embraced traditional medical practices such as herbal medicine with fervour. The increasing acceptance of alternative therapies marks a profound change in attitude towards health and the body. This has resulted in a significant proliferation of alternative and complementary therapy practitioners as the disenchantment with modern drug therapy has increased. Moreover, the over-prescription of medication that can render drugs ineffective (eg. antibiotic resistance) has been a major contributory factor in the popularity of herbal remedies, as have the often numerous, unpleasant and undesirable side-effects experienced with large doses of synthetic drugs. Such trends in the West contrast with other parts of the world, such as the Caribbean, parts of Africa, regions of South America, India and China which have used herbal remedies as an integral way of living. It is in fact conventional medicine and modern medical thinking that is regarded with scepticism amongst such traditional cultures.

The fundamental difference lies in how illness and disease is viewed. Modern medicine emphasises the symptoms whereas traditional therapists such as medical herbalists adopt a more holistic approach to diagnosis and treatment, considering aspects of the patient's circumstances and the context in which they have fallen ill. This has proved more successful than conventional medicine in cases where certain conditions are mere manifestations of an underlying or deep-rooted cause.

An examination of the state of health in Western societies, show that despite the vast expenditure on health care, large numbers in the population remain relatively unhealthy. Chronic illnesses such as respiratory disorders, heart disease and diabetes are on the increase; approximately 50% of the population in Western countries are prescribed drugs for conditions as diverse as asthma, arthritis, depression and high blood pressure. Countries that practise Herbal Medicine (despite abject poverty, deprivation and limited resources for medical provision, not to mention climatic conditions that favour the spread of infection) remain relatively healthy by comparison. Physical ailments experienced so frequently in Western societies appear to be more symptomatic of age and decline in the poorer nations, rather than inherent health problems of a particular culture.

The preference for herbal alternatives over conventional medication in treating a wide variety of illnesses, either acute or chronic continues to remain a matter of choice in a culture of quick fixes and time constraints. Herbal treatments are more gentle remedies and usually take longer to have an effect than modern drugs.

(ii) Treating the 'whole person'

Conventional doctors are trained to make a clinical diagnosis based on symptoms and findings from an examination. Sometimes, tests are carried out that will make or confirm a diagnosis based on these initial findings. Treatment is based on these symptoms, clinical findings and the diagnosis. This has great value in certain medical conditions and we are living in an age of great medical and technological advancements. Due credit must be given to the great work that is done within conventional medical practices today.

However, most of us will see a GP for conditions that are probably preventable, recurring or chronic and so requiring a focus on managing the condition. Herbal Medicine, when incorporated can be used to prevent illness in the first instance by optimising health, for example, improving the immune function and so making it more robust at fighting infection. Equally, it can be an effective treatment in a number of acute and chronic conditions. The main difference in these two medical practices lies in how illness and disease is viewed. Modern medicine focuses on the symptoms whereas traditional therapists such as medical herbalists also consider the context in which illness has occurred. This also holds true for the treatment. Often, herbs are used as a preventative measure in fighting infection or illness and it is popularly used to enhance or maintain optimum health and well-being. The demand for natural ingredients over synthetic is evidenced by the vast array of herbal proprietary brands and products ranging from toiletries to herb teas and foods. Even the cosmetic industry is slowly gaining insight into the traditional beauty secrets of Africa and the far-east and other cultures that value natural plant products in skin care regimes.

The word holistic comes from the Greek work '*holos*' meaning whole. Viewing a person's illness in a holistic context is all about seeing them as a whole and not just focussing on the part of the body that is not working or is damaged. Taking into account a person's well-being must give due consideration to their psychological as well as their spiritual aspects of health. A holistic approach to physical problems would attempt to identify the cause(s) of the condition or illness having taken the initial steps to address the symptoms in order to alleviate any discomfort or pain. By taking a simple case history, the herbal practitioner will be able to gather the most important points regarding the patient and the outside influences which may be contributing to the illness. Examples of these factors could include bereavement, stress, divorce, work pressure (eg. staff appraisal, performance-related incentives), moving house etc... Some of the symptoms of stress and how it can affect our health has been explained briefly in Chapter 1. Stress-related disorders are numerous and diverse. Stress can affect each person in a unique manner and whilst some will cope remarkably under the most stressful situations, many others simply 'fall apart' displaying physical and mental signs and symptoms. The real purpose of holistic healing is to examine these factors in close detail but importantly, to see if there is a real discernable difference between these outside factors and a connection to illness compared to the signs and symptoms of mere organic disease.

Stress-related illness and the holistic diagnosis

Most people would not consider it 'rocket science' to work out that whatever factor is causing them stress (called the stressor) could also be making them ill. However, due to the body's remarkable capacity to cope with stress, this connection between the stressor and their symptoms is not always so glaringly obvious. Insidious and subtle manifestations are difficult to diagnose but very often, examining the wider influences on the person and identifying any contributory factors will make diagnosis and treatment that much more effective.

Symptom	Possible organic cause(s)	Likely stressor(s)
Headache	Eyesight problems, eyestrain through computer overuse & screen glare	Anxiety, worry
Sinusitis	Bacterial infection of the sinuses	Sinus congestion from reduced immune responses. Decreased resistance to infection can arise from persistent stress
Recurring colds	Virulent viral infection	Reduced immunity from prolonged or sustained stress
Palpitations	Early warning signs of heart disease	Anxiety (many outside factors)
High blood pressure	Dietary causes	Stress, anxiety
Skin disorders eg psoriasis	Immune disorder	Made worse through stress
Hair loss	Nutritional deficiency esp B vitamins, genetic (male pattern baldness), medication	Worry, anxiety, stress

Herbs and holistic healing

Strictly speaking, herbal medicine as it is practised in the West today is considered an alternative form of medicine. That is, herbal remedies are used instead of conventional drugs to treat or manage illness or medical conditions. However, the term 'alternative' used in this context can be sometimes be misleading and confusing because although it is often used instead of taking conventional drugs, it does not mean than herbs cannot be used to complement conventional medical treatment. In some cases, the use of herbal medicines can form the basis of adjunct therapy. That is, it can enhance the effectiveness of conventional treatments with results being more profound than with either therapy used on its own. However, herbal medicine as a complement to conventional drug treatment is quite rare because in reality, there are all sorts of issues with herb-drug interaction that does not permit this kind of practice. Equally, most people invariably seek herbal alternatives when their bodies do not respond readily to conventional drugs or they are opposed to taking strong drugs when they would rather try a more natural and effective alternative that has been used traditionally in other parts of the world for many years.

As mentioned earlier, much of the success in herbal medicine can be attributed to healing within a holistic context in as much as the effectiveness of the herbs themselves. The unique medicinal properties of a number of herbs will be discussed in more detail later on in the book. The symptoms of the current problem are addressed in relation to the whole person by examining the social and cultural context in which the illness has occurred and in which the healing process takes place.

Moreover, some herbal preparations (known as tonics) can be used to enhance and promote good health and vitality by maintaining essential body systems and their functioning at a peak. So, relatively 'healthy' individuals may choose to take herbal tonics for a short period of time to boost their immunity for example or to stave off a cold. Some may choose to take a tonic to improve their digestive function and to improve bowel movement. Others may choose to take a tonic to improve liver function or in improve circulation. The use of herbal tonics in this manner can be fundamental not only in maintaining a sense of well-being but more importantly, in preventing disease and illness. This does not mean that herbal tonics should replace a well balanced diet based on good nutritional practises. However, such tonics can promote the health and function of important organs and systems such as the liver, kidneys, circulation etc…. all of which optimise vital body functioning and getting the most from our diet. Herbal tonics can be a great supplement to a healthy well balanced lifestyle that would include things like adequate exercise, relaxation, recreational pursuits and hobbies, in addition to good nutrition. In essence though, herbal medicine is about restoring balance and its applications can be particularly effective in supporting the cleansing and detoxifying action of organs that are responsible for eliminating wastes from the body. This would involve the bowel, the kidneys, the skin and the lungs, all assisted by a healthy circulatory system.

The main focus of herbal medicine in the context of holistic healing is to provide treatments that will encourage the body to heal itself. This may involve a preparation of a single herb or a more commonly, a combination of herbs as many different areas may need to be targeted. The mechanisms for herbal action are not fully understood for all medicinal herbs although there is ample evidence on mode of action for some ingredients in some of the more popular herbs. This is the subject of much research in many countries worldwide including, the US, China, Germany and India as well as the UK. Since two thirds of conventional drugs are derived from plant origin. There is strong drive to develop new and effective drugs from plant sources. Research into more effective treatments is increasingly based on existing herbal cures in an attempt to discover new drugs. Those remedies that represent a long tradition of use in many parts of the world may ultimately hold the clue to finding a breakthrough cure for some of the more debilitating and destructive killer diseases of the 21st century such as cancer and AIDS.

The fundamental difference between conventional medicine and traditional herbal medicine lies very much in the treatment. Extensive research has shown that some medicinal plants used in their whole state have a greater therapeutic effect than the equivalent dosage of isolated active ingredients. It is widely believed that the natural combination of these key constituents in some whole plants works in synergy with each other, maximising their effectiveness and exerting a medicinal effect. This medicinal effect cannot be reproduced by one or more of the active ingredients on their own, as is so often preferred in conventional medicine. This is the basis of conventional drug treatment and although necessary in some instances where potency is the requirement, the side effects are very much the down side of this form of treatment.

This is not to say that commercial preparations of herbal supplements do not contain individual active constituents (AC). On the contrary since the more reputable brands are prepared from whole herbs in such a manner as to ensure that the preparation contains known quantities of the active ingredients. They have therefore been standardised to contain known levels of the active ingredients which has been shown to exert a therapeutic effect at the quantity specified. These preparations are often labelled and marketed as 'standardised extracts' and many people find this a convenient and effective way to take herbal medicines. The more traditional herbalists would subscribe to the notion that standardised is getting away from whole herb preparations and in some cases, moving away from traditional practices. Both forms are effective and the varying viewpoints are very much dictated by the differing opinions of practitioners, the patients and the relationship between the two. Ultimately, the healing process is the most important factor here and a successful outcome is strongly influenced by what the patient best responds to, depending on his or her constitution in addition to the condition being treated.

(iii) A brief history of herbal medicine and cultural contexts of practice

The development of herbal medicine and its practice throughout the world has a strong history, with each country forming its own tradition of herbal pharmacy. This has become incorporated into its culture and what is unique to each tradition has developed through many years of knowledge, skill and practice. Some of the older traditions remain very much intact throughout history and herbal medicine here continues to be practised in a manner of their ancestors and passed on through generations of healers.

Western herbal medicine as it is today is largely influenced by such history but is also influenced by other practices from other traditions through travel, folklore, colonisation and settlement. The relatively recent revival of herbal medicine in the West is really from the back of a decline in interest, partly due to the reputation and associations it once had with witches and witchcraft, astrology, mystical spirits and magical powers. Fortunately, modern science and drug development and the need to find new cures reignited interest in some of the traditions as well as to explore the rapidly expanding field of phytopharmacology (study of how plant chemicals can exert an influence in the body) and phytochemistry (study of the chemical constituents of plants, particularly medicinal herbs) in addition to current developments in modern medical science. Modern herbal medicine in the West is now very much a science and the art of good practice is to fully understand and respect these traditions as well as to respect the potency of some of the greatest medicinal herbs to benefit mankind.

Putting all this into context, it is important to start at the beginning and to examine the earliest records of how herbal medicine all began. Wild plants have been used for food and medicines long before records were kept. Medicinal and other uses were undoubtedly uncovered by trial and error, which may not have always been pleasant with probably some disastrous and tragic consequences for some. The plants explored would have been mainly native to the country at first before any 'foreign' species being cultivated in herb gardens specifically for the medicinal use (the basis for some of the commercial business now). Establishing when all this began is somewhat difficult since early documented evidence of medicinal use is sparse.

The earliest indication of herbal medicine is suggested from Babylonian records dating as far back as 2000BC which gives instructions for the preparation and administration of medicinal herbs. After that, the ancient Egyptians, renowned for their skills in embalming, started recording the use of herbal remedies on papyrus paper as early as 1600BC. Much of this is still in evidence today with a strong industry in distillation of perfume and medicinal oils as well as other notable products. Some of the herbs of that time included juniper, thyme and fennel, all of them used in Western herbal medicine today.

Other parts of the world like China, India and Native America were developing their own herbal practice, some of which survive to this day. China (Traditional Chinese Medicine or TCM) and India (Ayurveda) have the oldest written traditions, dating from around 1000BC. Some of the traditions of the Native Americans (Shamanism) have sadly been lost due to the European settlers who colonised the land. Much of the herbal knowledge that was passed on through generations by word of mouth rather than by a written record of it was wiped out through war and destruction. It is known however that these traditional practices were less scientific and influenced by a belief in magical powers, spirits and rituals. In some rural parts of South America, shamanism is still widely practised and there continues to be great interest within modern science to research into some of the medicinal benefits of certain indigenous plants especially of the rainforests.

In Australia, some aspects of traditional herbal medicine practice still exist in the native Aborigine culture although much of original traditions and knowledge has been lost due to the invasion of the European settlers. In a similar manner to Shamanism, the Aborigines believed that certain spirits held the power over health and disease. Much of this belief system continues to exist in their culture and ritualistic practices of today and though this is less scientific, the native Aborigines have extensive knowledge of the landscape and the indigenous plants of Australia, particularly those possessing medicinal properties.

The history of African herbal medicine has solid foundations in the traditional healers of the time passing on vital information about indigenous plants and those used as medicinal herbs. Most of this information was heavily influenced by the Middle—East and India which had an established trade for more than 3000 years. Again, colonial conquests wiped out much of this foundation knowledge and what remains has been misrepresented or replaced by Western medical principles for solutions to healthcare and hygiene. Traditional practices were not permitted to evolve or flourish. The demonisation of the African traditional approach is supported by the notion that much of it is dominated by voodoo and witchcraft, so much so that even the African people themselves have become somewhat distanced from it. Equally, it could be argued that in much of rural Africa, medical provision is sparse and not accessible to high tech services of modern hospitals and clinics. There is a heavy reliance on such traditions and use of medicinal herbs for many of the common disorders and diseases. Despite this however, in certain parts of Africa, the implementation of health programmes and initiatives from the West have modernised healthcare provision even though the ancient magical and spiritual beliefs of herbal traditions are still evident. As a consequence, what remains today is the coexistence of herbal practitioners who work closely with conventional doctors. It is probably one of those uncommon situations where the integrated approach to healthcare is best illustrated. With modern scientific influences, we are slowly becoming informed about the medicinal uses of the plants that have been used for centuries in Africa and finally understand how they work in curing illness and disease.

Herbal medicine in most of the Caribbean islands originates from the African traditions who brought their practices to the islands during the slave trade. This has survived as part of their long history and herbal medicine continues to be practised as a inherent part of their culture and tradition. Many of the Caribbeans have a high respect for this form of medicine. Herbal knowledge and skill is not confined to the healers or medical practitioners. The most notable herbal practitioners from the Caribbean was a Jamaican woman called Mary Seacole (1805-1881), a pioneering nurse and inveterate traveller who brought her skills as a nurse and herbal healer to the battlefields of the Crimean war to treat the sick and injured British soldiers. Using her own unique herbal formulations and remedies passed on through generations of traditional African healers, she became a real heroine of the war, along with her English counterpart, Florence Nightingale.

The Greeks also have a long tradition in herbal medicine, influenced by considerable knowledge on their cultivation and use. Around 400BC, Hippocrates (the 'father of medicine') lists a number of herbs with medicinal properties and makes many recommendations for his patients. The Ancient World honoured Hippocrates as the father of medicine because he considered all aspects of health and illness, some of which form the basis of conventional medicine as it is practised today. This is very much supported by scientific reasoning, research and evidence. Even medical students including qualified practitioners of herbal medicine honour Hippocrates by taking the 'Hippocratic Oath' upon completion of their training to signify a rite of passage as a practitioner of healing, whether conventional or herbal.

The Roman invasion resulted in the spread of herbal medicine in the regions and lands that they conquered because they brought with them the knowledge and uses of the healing plants. As many as 200 different species of herbs may have been introduced to Britain as a result of the Roman influence. This period also witnessed the influential work by the Greek physician Galen (130AD) who characterised medical wisdom at that time with his theories on the humors: *"In men, all diseases are caused by bile and phlegm. Bile and phlegm give rise to diseases when they become too dry or too wet or too hot or too cold in the body"*. This was later referred to as Galenical medicine and together with the incorporated wisdom of the Arab practitioner Avicenna (980-1037) formed the basis of conventional medical practices throughout the Middle Ages. After the collapse of the Roman Empire, much of the herbal knowledge and practice in Europe was sadly lost but what remained was continued by the Christian monks who grew herbs in their gardens that were attached to their monasteries. This is still very much in evidence today in some of the rural French and Italian monasteries. Physicians such as Paracelcus (1493-1541), marked their own individual stamp on the practice of herbal medicine on the whole. At this time, herbal remedies were very much part of medicine per se and most physicians were also alchemists. They therefore had great skill in investigating natural substances including plant materials and transforming them. They practised this with an early philosophical and spiritual discipline, combining elements of chemistry, metallurgy, physics, medicine, astrology, semiotics (study of human communications especially signs and symbols), mysticism, spiritualism and art.

The period of the Renaissance and the New World were exciting times for herbal medicine which saw the application of a more scientific approach to the study of herbs and medicinal plants. They were periods in time that were hugely influential in shaping the knowledge and practice of Western Herbal Medicine as it is today. Key players such as the English astrologer and physician Nicholas Culpepper (1616-54) and the American herbal practitioner Samuel Thomson (1769-1843) were instrumental in making herbal medicine more accessible to the common people rather than it being exclusive to the elite rich and upper classes. Equally, travellers to and from other parts of Europe, the Americas and the rest of the world also influenced the cross-fertilisation of herbal knowledge between countries, traditions and cultures.

The decline of herbal medicine from the late 18th century saw the persecution of 'witches' who came to be synonymous with the practice of witchcraft, the possession of evil spirits, magical powers and the use of herbs. This reputation became hard to shift and coincided with the development and rapid progress of allopathic (conventional) medicine. Modern drug therapy however, is really based on this strong history of herbal medicine (as outlined above) and the study of the chemical constituents of medicinal herbs. Many of the common drugs are synthetic versions or derivatives originating from natural plant chemicals. Examples include aspirin (from salicylic acid extracted from the bark of the willow tree), the chemotherapy drugs vincristine and vinblastine (from the Madagaskar periwinkle herb). Vinblastine is mainly useful for treating Hodgkin's disease, advanced testicular cancer and advanced breast cancer. Vincristine is mainly used to treat acute leukemia and other lymphomas. Another anticancer drug, taxol is from the yew tree and the heart drug digitoxin is from the foxglove. More recently however, there has been a revival of herbal medicine as the long-term effects of conventional drugs is being realised in addition to the unpleasant side-effects of some of the more potent drugs. The gentle nature of herbal remedies and the holistic context in which it is practised is very much in favour as an increasing number of people are becoming disenchanted with modern drug treatments. This is especially the case for conditions that are preventable and are minor and particularly appealing if a natural form of therapy can be more effective in some instances.

(iv) Prevention, Cure and Herbal Medicine

The impact of any illness can have far-reaching consequences with psychological and emotional effects than just the mere physical unpleasantness that is experienced. Efforts being made by the various organisations and professional bodies through the implementation of health initiatives and programmes to adopt healthier lifestyles has emphasised the importance of prevention in as much as addressing specific health problems. Good health means different things to different people but we can all find ways of improving our quality of life which includes the prevention of minor illnesses through to the onset of major disease.

Many of the ailments and conditions often experienced by so many are simply symptomatic of age and decline. Age-related disorders are often unavoidable as much as the ageing process itself which increases the risk of age-related conditions (eg. arthritis, memory loss etc...). However, with sensible precaution and preventative measures which promote the maintenance of good health and vitality, the risk of onset of many of these conditions can be minimised and delayed. Importantly, the progression onto major disease can be significantly reduced by taking appropriate measures that reduce their risk.

The factors that influence illness are as diverse and numerous as the variety of diseases themselves. Cultural differences have highlighted the need for a deeper understanding of the person and the context in which they have fallen ill. This encapsulates not only the holistic philosophy of treating illness but it also demonstrates the immense power of the mind over body concept in addition to the outside influences that determine onset and progression of disease. This is not to say that addressing the physical manifestations of illness is less important, far from it. However, clear links between the mind and body illustrates the equal importance of the attitudes towards ill-health and the psychological approaches that are necessary for total recovery.

To change attitudes, whatever the issue is by no means an easy task. To assert positiveness despite overwhelming factors that engulf the mind, way of thinking, feeling, behaving and functioning seems almost impossible. However, time and time again, there have been numerous examples of how a change in attitude and way of thinking has led not only to radical improvements in the quality of life but in some instances, the beginning of the recovery process in illness. Preventing illness can be achieved by ensuring a well-balanced diet, adequate exercise and adopting healthy lifestyle choices. Anything that is not promoted as a 'healthy choice' for eg. alcohol, can be taken in moderation and very little at that. Many people have a tendency to be lazy. The temptation is to eat all the tasty foods (invariable those that are considered bad for you) and do as little exercise as possible. To compound matters, most people want quick fixes and get into bad habits with diet and exercise. Poor habits from a young age is also an important element since many of the taste patterns for food and lifestyle choices are determined pretty early on in life and much of my work as a herbalist is really to educate the parents on fundamentals of good nutrition and healthy lifestyles in order to prevent the pattern of poor habits being passed on to their children.

In respect of maintaining optimum health and vitality, the following aspects describe how herbal medicine can assist, particularly in preventing illness and disease. Herbs have demonstrated their immense medicinal value not only in the treatment of disease but also in maximising health and well-being. Such 'herbal tonics' as they are referred to, can be incorporated quite simply into a daily routine or as part of a specific health regime. . Moreover, herbal tonics may be individually formulated depending on the part of the body requiring special attention eg. kick-starting a sluggish liver or improving digestive function. Tonics may also be taken for general aid to gently invigorate the body systems. Such preventative measures are becoming quite popular and coincides directly with the increasing demand and sale for natural health products and herbal supplements. Tonics may serve the purpose of maintaining body systems in optimum condition such as:

a) Revitalising and body conditioning
b) Detoxification
c) Elimination
d) Boosting immunity/increasing resistance to infection

Revitalising and body conditioning

Taking herbal tonics is a gently way in which the body systems are strengthened, toned and enlivened, ensuring their peak functioning. The whole body can benefit as well as individual systems that require special attention. In this instance, specific herbs can be prescribed, for eg. kick-starting a sluggish liver into action or tonics to improve digestive function in order to enable the body to make the most from nutrients from the diet, or indeed to extract the essential nutrients from the food itself. Moreover, tonics such as these will enable the body to utilise the energy far more efficiently consequently improving body functioning on the whole. Additional areas for consideration in revitalising the body would be to examine the nervous system (which also includes mood, emotion and thinking), the circulation and immune function.

Important aspects of Western Herbal Medicine

Diet & Lifestyle
The importance of good nutrition cannot be sufficiently emphasised. Many of the disorders, illnesses and diseases witnessed today in modern society can be directly linked to poor dietary practices, often prolonged or in severe cases, malnutrition.

The herbalists' approach to treatment or management of any condition will invariably consider aspects of the patient's diet, very often in some detail. Nutritional Therapy is fast gaining value as an important tool in tackling symptoms of modern living, in addition to ensuring optimum nutrition for all individuals.

Lifestyle choices can have a significant impact on health and well-being. In aiming to address symptoms within a holistic framework, herbalists invariably consider the lifestyle choices of the patient in addition to suggesting changes or areas for improvement. Factors such as smoking, alcohol consumption, lack of exercise, work patterns, stress management, recreational pursuits etc.... are all aspects of lifestyle that is considered in some detail. In advising patients of a work-life balance, herbalists often consider the lifestyle choices of their patients and try to advise of modifications, particularly where it has been shown to be inexorably linked to their symptoms.

Detoxification

Toxins are poisons which manifest in the body at varying levels of potency. They are constantly introduced into the body through the food that is consumed, through the air and through water.

Additionally, our bodies also produce a variety of toxins as waste products or as by-products of the various metabolic processes. Gradual build up of these unwanted, and quite simply, poisonous substances can lead to ill-health (infection) or even disease. Despite this onslaught of toxicity, the body has a remarkable capacity to detoxify such toxins, that is, to break them down in such a manner that they become either less toxic to the body, or are converted into innocuous substances that are eventually excreted. The role of the liver is fundamental in keeping the toxins in the blood at a minimum level such that we remain illness-free. The immune system is also a key player in this detoxification process, as are the circulatory systems that assist in the removal of the toxins to the excretory organs. In this respect, the blood and lymphatic system are vital systems in supporting the crucial role of the liver and associated detoxifying organs in maintaining optimum health. Herbal tonics that revitalise these organs help a great deal, especially if they have been neglected (through poor diet, or damage). This particularly applies to the liver since it is the first port of call for detoxifying any toxic substances that have entered the body (through the gut or via the bloodstream).

Toxic build up is an inevitable part of all metabolic processes that occur in the body, although the liver's ability to make them less harmful is very impressive. In this respect, it is worth noting, not the actual number of times we fall ill but in fact, the periods of time in which we remain symptom-free. Without this vital function we will continually suffer illness and disease. Poor dietary habits over a long time can impair the vital detoxifying function of the liver and some of the more harmful substances that we consume (like alcohol and prescription drugs) can even damage the liver cells, making them less able to cope over time. This explains why so many with poor diets and lifestyles are perpetually run down, lacking in energy, have lost their vitality and are prone to infections. Herbs which are notable in assisting the functions of the liver are dandelion (*Taraxacum officinale*), milk thistle (*Silybum marianum*) and fringetree (*Chionanthes virginicus*) amongst others. Some of these herbs are commonly included in herbal tonics for this particular purpose. Equally, they are also prescribed by herbalists for conditions that have a metabolic basis.

The eastern philosophy of fasting is now also commonly practised by some in the West as an active choice in adopting a healthier lifestyle. Some of the world's major religions such as Hinduism, Buddhism and Islam have well established traditions in fasting and with scientific knowledge, it now appears that regular fasting is an effective way of cleansing the system of toxins and optimising health & well-being. Provided that it is done sensibly, vital body systems, particularly the digestive system, the liver and the kidneys have an opportunity to rest, preventing not only their exhaustion (when illness can set in) but eliminating any potentially infective agents that are lying dormant within the systems.

Herbs for Detox

Much has been written about and publicised on the subject of detox and detox diets. Commercial interest must be viewed with some caution and much of what passes for 'detox' is simply good nutrition, sensible eating combined with a healthy lifestyle.

Considering the amount of 'invisible' toxins in the environment, common medications, lifestyle habits and toxins consumed in food, it is perhaps easy to see how almost everyone in a Western society can expect to suffer from some degree of toxicity. In the worse case scenario, the toxic burden on these vital organs has been known to be a major contributory factor for some forms of cancer, particularly cancer of the bowel.

The body has its own natural detoxifying organs: the liver, the kidneys, the digestive system and associated organs and structures. The elimination of toxins from our cellular environment, including those from foods must consider the efficient functioning of all these organs systems in addition to a good circulatory system. Proper nutrition, a well balanced diet and a healthy lifestyle are all factors that will assist this process and prevent toxic overload on these vital structures.

Our diet has a very important part to play in detoxification. Consequently, what we consume can assist our organs and there is some excellent literature on the foods that are recommended for this purpose (*see recommended reading at the end*).

I focus on the liver here as it is central to 'detox'. It is essential to appreciate that the health of the liver is directly dependent on the type and quality of the food that is consumed. Though it carries out essential detoxification, like any other vital organ, it has its own nutritional requirements in order to perform its function of repair, regeneration and rebuilding.

In a nutshell, foods to cut out are those that are rich in refined sugars (such as cakes, biscuits, chocolates, sweets etc…), pre-prepared or ready-made meals, foods containing hydrogenated and trans fats, alcohol and drugs (including tobacco). Examples of the kinds of foods that are beneficial to the liver in its health and hence, its proper function are listed below. These include plenty of fresh fruit and vegetables.

FRUITS		**VEGETABLES**	
Lemons	Contains an important chemical which assists in the breakdown of gallstones. Also contains pectin, a soluble form of fibre which is good for bowel health (prevents constipation) and lowers blood cholesterol. A good source of vitamin C too	Artichoke	Helps reduce cholesterol and other fats in the blood. Improves the detoxification, repair and regeneration capacity of the liver. Also protects against liver damage
Apples & Oranges	Both contain pectin which prevents constipation. Also helps reduce cholesterol in the blood. Apple contains a host of important nutrients incl. antioxidants which can help protect against cancer. Oranges are a good source of vitamin C	Brussels sprouts	Part of the brassica family (other examples are cabbages, turnips, broccoli, cauliflower and swedes) so helps in the detoxification processes of the liver. Increases oestrogen metabolism and excretion so thought to confer protection against some of the oestrogen-dependent cancers, particularly breast and uterine cancer
Grapes	Excellent for preventing heart disease (contains important chemicals called proanthocyanidins) which are also antioxidants so will help prevent cancer as well	Cabbage & turnip	Cabbage, one of the oldest of the brassicas, and the ancestor of broccoli and cauliflower. Cabbage, like other brassicas, is high in sulphur, so excellent for liver health. Helps in the detoxification processes and confers protection against cancer through its antioxidant activity. Similar benefits from consuming turnips but both the leaves and root need to be eaten.
Pineapple & Papaya	Both contain naturally-occurring enzymes that help breakdown protein from food so will help digestion. Also contains cancer preventing antioxidants	Broccoli	Broccoli, another popular member of the brassica clan has similar benefits to the liver
Grapefruit	Contains important nutrients, antioxidants and pectin. A key player in liver detox reactions	Leeks	Highly nutritious and contains key antioxidants such as the bioflavonoids. Also contains sulphur compounds which assist in the detoxification role of the liver
Berries esp	Contain high levels of	Watercress	Rich in the antioxidant beta-carotene.

dark red, blue or black	proanthocyanidins and bioflavonoids that help protect against major diseases like heart disease and cancer also contains other important nutrients such as vitamin C and carotenes (both have antioxidant properties)		Also contains sulphur. Both are excellent for the liver

Herbs and spices are also beneficial to the liver. Some of the more common ones which are great in any detox programme include the following:

Garlic
Onions
Fennel
Radish
Dandelion

More on good nutrition later in the book.

Therapeutic agents in the biotransformation of toxins

The body's ability to make toxic substances less toxic or harmless to the body is referred to as biotransformation. The liver is critical in this function and contains key enzymes which break down these poisonous by-products of metabolism (or metabolites) and convert them into harmless substances. Part of this biotransformation process involves a key enzyme system in the liver known as the cytochrome P_{450} enzyme system, which is found in the liver. Another key liver enzyme in this regard is known as glutathione S-transferase (or GST for short). In fact, the liver function tests that are carried out to assess liver function often determine levels of these key enzymes as an indicator of liver damage, disease or dysfunction. Any herb that can support the liver in boosting the biotransformation processes will indirectly assist in detoxification. Hepatics are herbs that promote liver function but can also protect lever cells from harmful toxins or indeed repair liver cells once damage has already occurred.

Schisandra chinensis (schisandra)↑ glutathione status ie. induces GST activity. Contains 2 key active constituents (Schisandrin B and Gomasin A). They have the following characteristics:

- Schisandrin B   - ↑ microsomal cytochrome P_{450} enzymes
                     - ↑ GST activity

- Gomasin A   - ↑ bile acid synthesis & metabolism
                     - stimulates liver regeneration
                     - ↑ GST activity

Curcuma longa (turmeric)
- Chemopreventive of carcinogenesis (alters the activation/detoxification of carcinogen metabolism)

Silybum marianum (milk thistle)
- Protects intact liver cells that have not yet been irreversibly damaged by preventing the entry of toxins through their cell membranes (acts on the cell membranes themselves)
- Stimulates protein synthesis thereby accelerating the process of liver cells regeneration and production of new cells

Culinary Herbs and Foods

Rosemary and **Sage** contain CARNOSOL which has antioxidant properties ie. it induces important liver enzymes (GST and NADPH-quinone reductase)

Garlic - chemoprotective against carcinogenesis
- induces liver activity (biotransformation)

Parsley leaf oil contains MYRISTICIN which induces GST activity

Citrus fruit oil increases GST activity

Green tea - contains POLYPHENOLS which are chemoprotective against carcinogenesis
- increases liver enzyme activity
- blocks cigarette-induced genetic damage in cells. Chromosomal or genetic damage can result in abnormal cell proliferation & differentiation – a classic hallmark of malignant change

The Brassicas   eg. brussel sprouts, cabbage, broccoli, horse radish
Contain GLUCOSINOLATES (S-glycosides)

upon cooking releases

ISOTHIOCYNATES
(contain sulphur)

1. cancer-preventing properties
2. anti-cancer properties
3. ↑ GST (liver & small intestine) in men only
4. specifically protective against colon cancer

Some herbs are particularly useful for the 3 key organs involved in detoxification:

The Liver: Dandelion – root & leaf
Milk Thistle
Beetroot
Red clover
Fennel
Green tea
Lemon and Lime
Carrots
Tomatoes

The Gut (esp colon):   Green leafy vegetables
Bio-yoghurt
Figs, Prunes, Dates
Olive Oil
Porridge

The Kidneys: Water (and plenty of it!!)
Grapefruit
Flaxseeds
Walnuts
Blueberries
Soy beans

Weight Loss regimes and Herbal Medicine

There is no substitute for a well balanced diet combined with adequate exercise and a healthy lifestyle. There are no wonder drugs or herbs for reducing weight. The popularity of some herbal supplements as slimming aids has some basis if viewed in context with a broader and more sensible weight loss regime. However, some of the herbs are extremely potent and can have adverse reactions and side-effects. They must be taken with caution and with advice from a medical herbalist.

Ephedra sinica (Ephedra or ma huang)

Ephedra, also known as ma huang, is a strong stimulant and found in some popular weight loss supplements. Despite it's widespread use in over-the-counter weight loss pills, there is no firm evidence that it promotes weight loss. Ephedra reduces appetite and stimulates fat metabolism, making it very effective as a weight-loss supplement. The active compound in Ephedra (*Ma Huang*) is ephedrine. Ephedrine increases the metabolic rate, so that your body burns fats and sugar more efficiently. By mobilising stored fat and carbohydrate reserves, ephedrine reduces appetite.

However, the Food and Drug Administration (FDA) in the US has received over 800 reports linking ephedra with dizziness, headaches, chest pain, psychosis, seizures and strokes. It has been previously banned by the FDA in some states and restricted for sale in the UK. This is because when ephedra is taken regularly in weight loss supplements, your body stays in an unnaturally high gear and there is risk for heart palpitations and heart attacks.

In the UK, the sale of ephedra is already restricted so products containing less than 1,800 milligrams can only be sold following a consultation with a herbal medicine practitioner.

Products containing higher doses of ephedra can only be sold in pharmacies.

Yerbe Maté (*Ilex paraguariensis*)

Yerbe Maté is a tea derived from the South American holly tree (*Ilex paraguariensis*) with a long tradition of use in Native America. It has only recently been marketed commercially in the West as a stimulant, dietary supplement and as an aid to weight loss owing to its reputed property as an appetite suppressant. The dried leaves are brewed and taken as a daily stimulant to invigorate the mind and body as well as a promoter of optimum health.

Yerbe Maté possesses a plethora of health benefits from being a rich source of important nutrients to its effects on the immune system, cardiovascular system, nervous system and gut. It contains polyphenolic compounds that exert very powerful antioxidant properties thus conferring protection against disease and cancer. Its most popular use is as a stimulant in weight loss by promoting thermogenesis (generating heat through the breakdown of fat stores) and as an appetite suppressant. It is taken as a suitable alternative to coffee and ordinary tea, and like them, is a diuretic.

The most notable active constituent in Yerbe Maté is mateine, a xanthine compound of which caffeine is another. The effects of mateine are more desirable than any of the related compounds since it exhibits the best combination of xanthine properties without side effects. It is an effective bronchodilator and therefore very useful in asthma. It stimulates the CNS (central nervous system) without being addictive and induces better attributes of sleep. It also relaxes peripheral blood vessels being clinically beneficial in reducing blood pressure.

As an alternative to coffee, Yerbe Maté is the preferred choice since observational studies show that it produces similar, if not, better clinical effects without the undesirable side effects that accompany most natural stimulants. Limited clinical trials have been conducted on this herb, and therefore its effectiveness is unclear but there has been much interest shown in North America in the last decade since its commercial marketing. Exceeding recommended doses can increase the risk of oesophageal cancer due to the high binding capacity of the tannins and polyphenols in the tea.

Hoodia gordonii (Asclepiadaceae family)

Hoodia gordonii has been used by the South African San tribe for thousands of years who used it when they went on long hunting expeditions. Hoodia helped to prolong their hunting trips by suppressing hunger, and increasing their energy levels.

There are various species of Hoodia but the *gordonii* variation is the only one that contains the natural appetite suppressant. Hoodia pills kills the appetite and attacks obesity, is organic with no synthetic or artificial appetite control agents and has no side effects. Researchers have identified the active ingredient as P57, which suppresses the appetite. P57 is currently being considered for marketing as a commercial slimming pill.

Hoodia is a natural substance that literally takes your appetite away. Aside from using it to stop hunger, it provides unperturbed energy and combats stress. The San also use it to treat diabetes and hypertension. It's even said to cure hangovers and upset stomachs too.

Some manufacturers claim that when Hoodia is combined with a healthy eating plan and exercise, it can help to bring about tremendous changes in body fat, and can greatly improve a person's health.

Double blind clinical trials have not yet been completed with Hoodia. Even those interested in trying Hoodia without waiting for clinical trials to be completed may have difficulties, since Phytopharm®, the only licensed producer of Hoodia as a weight loss aid, does not yet market the product. Any other brands need to be viewed with caution since the relative scarcity of Hoodia means that the ingredient is hard for manufacturers to acquire. It is therefore hard to imagine how dozens of firms now claim to sell weight loss supplements containing Hoodia. There is as yet no conclusive evidence that Hoodia is a safe and effective appetite suppressant.

Elimination

Prevention of illness is also dependent upon the adequate elimination of waste products and toxins within the body. Organs that are instrumental in this function are the gut and the kidneys as well as the skin and the lungs but to a lesser extent. The blood has a secondary, yet vital role in assisting the main organs of excretion. Poor functioning of these organs (and systems) of elimination can not only affect health and well-being but more importantly, be symptomatic of a more serious underlying disorder. This does not even venture anywhere towards mentioning the complications that could arise from dysfunction in these organ systems. Toxic build up to abnormal proportions has damaging consequences for the body.

Herbs that can enhance the elimination function of the body include all the herbal laxatives which will work directly on the bowels. They vary in potency and are chosen carefully depending on the severity of the problem being treated. However, long-term prescription of herbal laxatives is not usually common practice since prescription of any herbal medicines will be accompanied by comprehensive dietary advice, modifications and recommendations. Notable herbal laxatives such as senna (*Cassia senna*), rhubarb (*Rheum palmatum*) and buckthorn bark (*Rhamnus frangula*) are very useful in enhancing the elimination process in the gut and herbal diuretics such as celery (*Apium graveolens*) can be added to most herbal tonics. They serve an important purpose in achieving the main objective in preventative medicine.

Boosting immunity/increasing resistance to infection

Additional benefits of herbal tonics include the assistance and support of the body's natural defence mechanisms in the fight against infection and disease. Many would have heard of Echinacea (*Echinacea purpurea*) although its effectiveness is yet to be proved. Despite this, many have sought relief from the common cold in addition to preventing the onset of it. Its ability to do this has been postulated and a number of theories exist on its immune enhancing properties although endorsement from the medical profession is still not forthcoming. In contrast, many doctors and healthcare professionals have a high regard for garlic (*Allium sativum*), not only in boosting immune defences and combating infection but also in its cardiovascular and circulatory benefits. There is a significant body of evidence to prove its effectiveness for a number of conditions and as a prophylactic supplement. The holistic approach to treatment is to enhance and improve the body's own immune responses, thereby enabling the body to rely on its own system to resist infection rather than resorting to a heavy reliance on conventional drugs as a combative measure.

Additionally, other herbs are also useful in combating infection such as the ginsengs (Korean and Siberian ginseng, *Panax ginseng* and *Eleutherococcus senticosus* respectively) but they are probably more renowned for their tonic and strengthening properties rather than as anti-infective herbs. Equally, diet is fundamental in maintaining a healthy immune system so ensuring adequate intakes of crucial micronutrients is strongly advised, for eg. vitamin C. The current recommended dietary intake for vitamin C is 90 mg for men and 75 mg for women (add an extra 35 mg for smokers). There is no credible evidence to suggest that megadoses of vitamin C improves health although a daily intake of 200 to 300 mg would be ideal. A good diet or a standard multivitamin can achieve this easily. The trace mineral zinc is another nutrient that is important in boosting immunity. A recommended daily intake of 15mg should be more than adequate and any dose larger than 25mg may cause anaemia and copper deficiency. It is strongly recommended that professional advice and assistance from either a medical herbalist or a clinical nutritionist is sought prior to any self-medication on vitamin/mineral or herbal supplementation.

The gentle actions of herbs

The medicinal value of herbs is best illustrated by looking at the manner in which they affect the body. Compared to conventional drugs, herbal remedies are on the whole, very gentle on the body but only if taken sensibly, with proper advice from a medical herbalist. Equally, their therapeutic value is highlighted when combined with a good diet because this symbiotic relationship works on the basis that without a good diet, the herbs cannot be effective and without herbs, the body cannot derive the best nutrition from food. The gentle, yet effective nature of herbs has also minimised the side effects commonly experienced from conventional drugs which appeals to most people.

Herbal tonics by their very nature is made up of herbs with gentle actions. They target specific organs and systems in an attempt to carry out four of the important actions that constitute holistic health; that is revitalisation, detoxification, elimination and resistance to infection. The following gives common examples of herbs that can be used for each body system, and although not exhaustive by any means, it does provide a general guideline as to the types of herbs that are used to rejuvenate and tackle the body system in question.

Body System	Comment
Skin	The skin should be regarded as an organ in itself as it carries out a number of important functions. Herbs such as cleavers, nettle and red clover gradually restore proper functioning of the skin to improve health and vitality.
Liver	Bitter tonics containing milk thistle, aloe or blue flag all aid the functioning of the liver. They tone and strengthen the organ as well as increasing the flow of bile into the digestive tract. This will enable a better breakdown of fats and prevent some of the more common problems associated with poor fat digestion.
Immunity	To combat minor infections, garlic and echinacea can be taken. For more resistant infections, more specific herbs such as goldenseal or barberry are good and bearberry is particularly good for urinary tract infections.
Nervous	Tonic remedies containing herbs such as skullcap, oats, St. John's Wort all assist the nervous system by toning and strengthening it. Science has a very difficult time of understanding what 'toning' and 'strengthening' means but in essence, the herbs either stimulate it or depress (relax) it thereby influencing their activity in this way. According to the condition being treated, herbs can target specific parts of the nervous system which exert control over a particular organ or system responsible for that condition. Most systems are affected by stress so some of the ginsengs particularly Siberian and Indian ginseng are particularly good at dealing with this.
Urinary	Various actions can be achieved by horsetail (astringent action of key constituents tighten and protect the main functioning part of the kidneys called the kidney tubules or nephrons). Other notable herbs can also help tone and strengthen the kidneys and

	associated structures such as cornsilk and bearberry both of which have diuretic properties. This will flush out any lingering toxins in the systems and prevent possible infection.
Digestive	Bitter tonics contain herbs that taste bitter (as the name implies) and via a reflex action involving the taste buds and automatic nerve control possibly to the brain, stimulate the digestive system (eg. to secrete more enzymes so that food can be better digested). Our digestive function declines with age and our diets need to be modified accordingly through the various life stages. Equally, there are other causes of poor appetite and digestion. It is critical to have good digestive function for all sorts of reasons, but mainly because we need to derive essential nutrients and energy. Restoring poor digestive function will help absorb vital nutrients and so prevent illness in this way. Herbs such as wormwood, gentian, dandelion and agrimony are all good at promoting digestive function in this way. Equally, bitter herbs such as bogbean, cumin and coriander are a good combination to increase appetite and stimulate digestion.
Respiratory	Poor respiratory function can leave a person prone to persistent coughs and colds. Build up of mucus (various causes) also increases the risk of chest infections so clearing this will be important in keeping this system functioning at its peak. Herbs such as elderflower and thyme are marvellous at working on this system as are elecampane, mullein and coltsfoot in clearing the chest of mucus.
Endocrine (hormonal)	This system covers a broad area and must be addressed specifically. For eg. Ginseng is good for stress and enabling the body to cope with it by adjusting to external pressures. It works directly on the adrenal glands (the organ responsible for producing adrenaline). Another example is the hormonally-active herb chaste berry (also known as agnus castus) which has a stimulating and normalising effect on the pituitary gland functions, in particular progesterone secretion. In this respect, it is often included in prescriptions for regulating the menstrual cycle and in PMS. However, because hormones cover such a wide spectrum, it is best to seek professional and comprehensive advice from a medical herbalist.
Heart & Circulation (Cardiovascular)	A number of different herbs have been attributed to improving the cardiovascular system which starts at the most important organ, the heart. Strengthening heart muscle can produce a more

	powerful heartbeat and blood can be pushed out more effectively. The heartbeat can also be regulated – Adonis (pheasant's eye or false hellebore) can be useful here. To improve localised and central circulation a number of herbs are useful including hawthorn berries, cayenne pepper, motherwort, ginger and ginkgo. For this system in particular, self-medication is not advised (not least because most of these herbs are not available for sale to the public) so a consultation with a medical herbalist is strongly recommended.
Musculo-skeletal	Joints and muscles require special attention, especially as we get older because of the risk of injury and symptoms that creep up due to wear and tear. To strengthen bones and connective tissue, horsetail, centella and comfrey can be used. To relax tense and cramped muscles, arnica, cramp bark or valerian can be used. Arnica is also known for its ability to reduce bruising. However, a consultation with a medical herbalist can identify specific areas for attention and they can prescribe the most suitable combination that is individually tailored.

Preventing illness – the cleansing action of herbs

Many advocates of alternative health measures believe that most illnesses can be avoided by not only adopting healthy lifestyles but that illness is caused by the inadequate removal of waste products and poor functioning of one or more of the body systems. Worse still, the longer it continues to malfunction, the greater the likelihood of toxins being reabsorbed back into the bloodstream and cells presenting a fresh challenge to the immune system and a whole new cycle of clearing the system of these substances begin. The cleansing action of specific herbs in eliminating such waste products and toxins have merit in being fundamental in the preventative measures taken to enhance and maintain optimum health and well-being.

The cleansing action of certain herbs on specific organ systems may take many forms but notably they are either eliminating, toning or defending. Each herb has a unique set of properties and actions all of which contribute to the overall health status of the person. The actions of such herbs can be briefly categorised as follows and described below.

Eliminating	Cleansing & Toning	Defence
Laxatives	Alteratives (deputatives)	Anti-microbials
Diuretics	Lymphatic tonics	Immune boosters
Diaphoretics	Other tonics	Diaphoretics
Expectorants	Adaptogens	

Elimination and Cleansing

Herb action	Definition	examples
Laxatives	Promotes increased bowel movement	buckthorn, rhubarb, senna
Diuretics	Stimulates the production & flow of urine	Celery, dandelion (leaf), cornsilk
Diaphoretics	Promotes sweating by the skin. Indirectly, they can also be useful in reducing fever by cooling the body down through increased sweating	Cayenne, angelica, boneset
Expectorants	Removes excess mucus from the respiratory system incl the lungs by stimulating coughing	Thyme, licorice, coltsfoot, white horehound, elecampane
Hepatics	Assists in the many functions of the liver incl its detoxifying role	Dandelion, milk thistle, *Schisandra* (Chinese magnolia vine)

Toning

Herb action	Definition	examples
Alteratives	Gradually restores balance to the body by working specifically on the areas out of balance which may be the cause of illness. Increases vitality and a good overall tonic for the body systems. Removes toxins from the cells and releases them into the bloodstream to be subsequently eliminated from the body. Accumulation of toxins leads to illness so its removal is vital to health	Yellow dock, red clover, nettles, heartsease, blue flag

	& well-being. This will gradually restore balance.	
Lymphatic tonics	Specifically promotes the healthy functioning of the lymphatic system (one of the systems involved in clearing the body of toxins)	Marigold, cleavers, burdock, echinacea
Specific tonics	Herbal formulations designed specifically to promote the healthy functioning of specific organs or systems	Specific herbs chosen for the organ or system being addressed
Adaptogens	Assists the body in coping with external pressures incl stress. They also support the normal functioning of body systems	Siberian ginseng, Indian ginseng

Defence

Herb action	Definition	examples
Anti-microbials	Combat infection directly by destroying the infective agent or inhibiting its effects within the body. Not all anti-microbial mechanism of action are fully understood	Garlic, goldenseal, wormwood, thyme, echinacea
Diaphoretics	Promoting the sweating process encourages the removal of the infective agents or their toxins through the skin	Boneset, cayenne, ginger all promote the sweating process
	Increased sweating can indirectly promote the cooling of the body and thus reduce fever. This will subsequently	Elderflower berries, peppermint, thyme, angelica

	eliminate infections	
Immune boosters	Boosts the body's natural defence mechanisms and protect the body against infection or disease	Siberian ginseng, wild indigo

CHAPTER 3 – MEDICINAL VALUE OF PLANTS

(i)   Actions of medicinal plants and herbs
(ii)   Home herbal pharmacy & herbal First Aid
(iii) Top 20 herbs – a guide to commercial preparations
(iv)   The role of the herbal medicine practitioner

(i) Actions of medicinal plants and herbs

The increasing popularity of herbal remedies may be attributed to two fundamental principles upon which this form of medicine works. Firstly, the concept of maintaining optimum health through incorporating herbal preparations into a daily routine; this gently enhances health and well-being and can prevent the onset of illness. Secondly, by providing herbal remedies or treatments which gently encourage the body to heal itself or by acting directly on the organs or tissues affected by illness and disease.

The quest to fully understand the mechanisms by which medicinal plants achieve this has fascinated scientists for many years and continues to this day through to modern medicine, research and development.

The significant evidence of successful treatment outcomes through the use of herbal remedies has created a need for a better understanding of <u>how</u> plant constituents/extracts exert their effect within the body. Specific actions of herbs may be due either to their individual chemical constituents or of equal importance, as is the case with most medicinal plants, the actions of the whole herb. In this respect, extensive study of such active constituents (AC) has demonstrated the presence of special characteristics or actions that are conferred to specific herbs and how they exert their actions by working in synergy with each other. The range of actions that are attributed to medicinal plants are briefly highlighted here.

The following is by no means exhaustive but merely a brief outline of the many actions of medicinal herbs and plants. The more common examples of herb actions are listed.

Herb action	Description	Common example(s)
Tonics	Herbs that will strengthen and tone specific parts of the body or whole organs to optimise their function	General tonics – the ginsengs (Siberian, Korean, Indian)
Laxatives	Herbs that work to promote the elimination function of the bowels by either increasing its motility or through providing bulk to the food eaten. Varying levels of strengths form aperients (v. mild) to cathartics and purgatives (v. strong)	Mild – goldenseal, dandelion (root) Stronger – senna, aloe Cathartic – buckthorn bark, senna Purgative – rhubarb

		Bulk laxative – flaxseed, psyllium husk
Diuretics	Herbs that promote the production of urine from the kidneys and its release from the bladder	Celery Dandelion (leaf)
Antiseptics	Herbs that counteract the potential impact of harmful organisms and so prevent illness	Garlic, tea tree oil juniper berries and bearberry (urinary tract antiseptic)
Antimicrobials	Herbs that will prevent the reproduction of infective, pathogenic organisms and so prevent illness	Garlic, goldenseal, tea tree, thyme, wild indigo, myrhh
Expectorants	Herbs that encourage the coughing up of mucus and phlegm from the chest and so prevent congestion and infection from getting worse	Thyme Licorice Wild Cherry, white horehound Elecampane
Antispasmodics	Herbs that counteract the effects of muscle spasms by either preventing or easing cramps. Considered as effective muscle relaxants too	Cramp bark Black haw Valerian root
Relaxants	Herbs that will calm and soothe the nervous system and particularly useful in anxiety states	Lemon balm Passion flower Chamomile
Sedatives and soporifics	Herbs that induce and regulate sleep	Valerian root Jamaica dogwood, lavender, wild lettuce
Hypnotics	Herbs that are stronger in their sedating action than sedatives or soporifics	Hops, Californian poppy Yellow jasmine
Anti-inflammatories	Herbs that reduce inflammation of affected areas. Can be applied internally or externally	Chamomile Marigold
Analgesics	Herbs that have pain-relieving properties	Willow (bark) Meadowsweet Yellow jasmine
Astringents	Tannin- containing herbs that promote the shrinking of tissues. In this way, they reduce secretions or discharges associated with illness	Witch hazel Oak Meadowsweet Agrimony

Bitters	Herbs that encourage appetite through indirect nervous stimulation of the brain via the gut (reflex action). Mechanisms of how this is achieved is poorly understood	Artemisia Gentian
Carminatives	Herbs that eliminate excess air and wind in the gut so reduce bloating and discomfort in the abdominal region	Peppermint, Sweetflag Cinnamon, Star anise Aniseed, Clove
Choleretics	Herbs that promote the production of bile from the liver. Bile is very important for the digestion of fats and can be useful in improving digestion	Barberry, Dandelion (root)
Cholagogues	Increases the secretion of bile from the gall bladder where it is stored. Promoting its secretion is just as important since poor digestion can be associated with poor secretion from the gall bladder despite production of it by the liver being normal.	Artichoke Fumitory Dandelion (root)
Demulcents	Herbs that soothe and protect inflamed or irritated internal tissues, linings such as mucous membranes of the gut, respiratory tract or the skin. Can be useful for external skin problems too	Licorice Mullein
Emollients	Herbs that provide a smooth covering to protect important linings especially mucous membranes	Marshmallow Slippery elm
Diaphoretics and sudorifics	Herbs that stimulate perspiration (sweating) thereby promoting the elimination of toxins through the skin.	Yarrow Elderflower
Emetics	Herbs that induce vomiting when taken in high doses. The action of emetics contribute to the overall cleansing and detoxification effect in illness that can be particularly beneficial to recovery	Lobelia (at excess doses). This is not an approach adopted by herbalists though many herbs taken in excess can induce vomiting
Anti-emetics	Herbs that prevent nausea and vomiting	Ginger, black horehound
Hepatics	Herbs that tone and strengthen the liver optimising its function	Milk thistle, schisandra
Nervines	Herbs that strengthen and tone the nervous system by either stimulating	St. John's Wort (antidepressant,

		certain nerve pathways (stimulants) or inhibiting others (relaxants)	anxiolytic), verbena (tonic), oats
Stimulants		Herbs that activate certain nerve pathways which quicken and enliven specific physiological functions	Rosemary Korean ginseng Ephedra (practitioners only)
Vulneraries		Herbs that promote healing, particularly of mucous membranes and skin	Marshmallow Centella, Comfrey, Chickweed
Emmenagogues		Herbs that have the ability to induce menstruation. They can work in a variety of ways, but the end result is menstruation. Its action can be mild or strong depending on the herb.	Chinese angelica Motherwort Blue cohosh Mugwort
Depuratives/ Alteratives		Herbs that promote detoxification by removing toxins and impurities from the cells, tissues and particularly the blood	Poke root Cleavers Blue flag
Styptics		Herbs that have the ability to stem external bleeding at the site of a wound or minor injury. They are applied topically to the localised area. Equally, for reproductive problems of haemorrhaging and very heavy bleeding during a period, they can be very useful	Shepherd's purse (♀) Lady's mantle (♀) Wild geranium (wounds) Horsetail (esp on urinary tract membranes)
Cardiotonics		Herbs that strengthen and tone the heart	Hawthorn, Motherwort
Circulatory stimulants		Herbs that promote the efficient functioning of the circulatory system by increasing blood flow to all parts of the body. Can work centrally (heart, lungs, gut, brain) or peripherally (skin and surrounding tissues)	Ginkgo Ephedra (practitioners only) Ginger Cayenne pepper

(ii) Home herbal pharmacy and herbal First Aid

For almost every medicine, there is a natural alternative. Symptoms of everyday ailments can be alleviated through using some of the following herbal remedies and preparations. For those who are keen to avoid a reliance on synthetic medications for commonly experienced problems or complaints, or more frequently, recurring ailments, it is always advisable to plan an 'alternative' medicine cabinet. A medicine chest stocked with herbal remedies for common ailments or for minor first aid can prove very useful, particularly for small children who, in my experience, respond extremely well to herbal alternatives. Herbal medicines have a proven record of combating symptoms the natural way and would certainly appeal to those concerned about some of the stronger conventional drugs with unpleasant side-effects. It is important to note that some of these herbal remedies have been passed on thorough generations, based on traditional knowledge and folklore that have stood the test of time and prove to be tried and tested remedies.

The home herbal pharmacy provides a plethora of gentle, yet effective alternatives for a wide variety of common ailments and minor injuries requiring some first aid. With the increasing availability of such pre-prepared herbal remedies on the market, the options are many. Some preparations have been specifically formulated from tried and tested herbal medicines that have a long history of effective use. Some are specific in their action eg. herbal cough mixtures, sleep remedies etc…

The following is a useful guideline into how a home herbal pharmacy can be planned, from a simple medicine chest to herbal First Aid. However, it is important to bear in mind that all medication (whether natural or conventional) should be taken with advice and some caution, and for any serious condition or injury that warrants emergency treatment, proper help should be sought without delay. <u>Never</u> mix herbal medicines with conventional drugs without proper advice from a qualified and registered practitioner of herbal medicine or a consultation with a doctor about the condition being treated. To compile your chest, it is advisable to seek the advice of a medical herbalist, especially on some of the more popular over the counter (OTC) medicines. The more expensive brands do not necessarily mean better quality of the product since they may be of very poor quality or limited in their therapeutic value (they may contain sub-therapeutic doses). Always ensure that your stock is within the best before date since the same applies to medicines as it does to food and never stock up more than you would need as some of the herbs may go rancid, particularly in a warm or humid environment. If in doubt, keep some of the liquid preparations in the fridge.

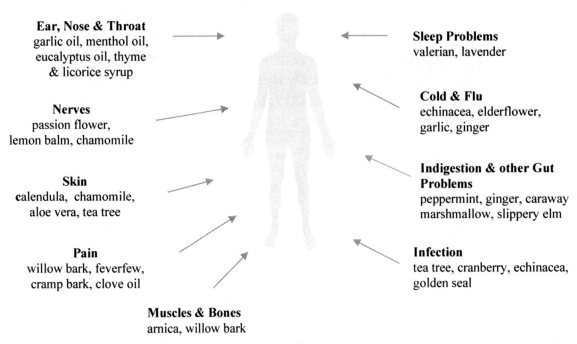

Ear, Nose & Throat
garlic oil, menthol oil,
eucalyptus oil, thyme
& licorice syrup

Nerves
passion flower,
lemon balm, chamomile

Skin
calendula, chamomile,
aloe vera, tea tree

Pain
willow bark, feverfew,
cramp bark, clove oil

Muscles & Bones
arnica, willow bark

Sleep Problems
valerian, lavender

Cold & Flu
echinacea, elderflower,
garlic, ginger

**Indigestion & other Gut
Problems**
peppermint, ginger, caraway
marshmallow, slippery elm

Infection
tea tree, cranberry, echinacea,
golden seal

THE MEDICINE CHEST (general use)

Colds and flu	Echinacea (best as a preventative treatment), ginger, elderflower tea, garlic
Sore throat, blocked nose, catarrh	Honey & lemon, oils of eucalyptus, menthol, peppermint and cajeput (inhalation), licorice
Coughs	OTC herbal cough syrups containing thyme, licorice, wild cherry bark
Indigestion & other digestive ailments (eg. bloating, acid indigestion/heartburn)	Peppermint oil, probiotics, tea made from caraway, aniseed and clove for indigestion. For heartburn, keep marshmallow tea or slippery elm tablets
Nausea, vomiting	Ginger (best as a tea). Also examine food intolerance issues if it's persistent
Sinus congestion	Inhalations of clove, menthol and eucalyptus oils
Headaches & migraines	Feverfew tablets, willow bark tablets
Toothache	Clove oil or cajeput oil (apply topically), willow bark tablets
Period pain	Cramp bark tablets, cypress and sage oils (topically)
Cystitis	Cranberry tablets, bearberry tablets, juniper berries (tablets or teas with all 3 herbs if symptoms are persistent or recurring)
Skin problems (eg. spots, pimples, rashes, allergic reactions)	Chamomile cream, calendula cream, lavender oil, tea tree lotion/oil
Earache, blocked ears or sinuses	Garlic oil, mullein, echinacea, goldenseal
Corns, verrucaes	Tea tree oil
Rheumatic aches & pains (muscular, joint)	Arnica gel/cream (topically), willow bark tablets,
Sleep problems (eg. Insomnia)	Valerian tablets/tea, lavender oil (inhalation)
Anxiety & stress	Passion flower & lemon balm (as tea), lavender oil (inhalation)
General pain	Willow bark tablets
Hangovers	Milk thistle tablets taken before a big night out, practical

	measures eg. increase water intake to prevent dehydration

CHILDREN'S MEDICINE CHEST

Headlice	Hair wash lotion containing tea tree oil, thyme oil
Cuts & grazes	Tea tree oil, Echinacea, herbal antiseptic cream containing lavender, eucalyptus and tea tree (be careful with broken skin & seek advice from a medical herbalist first)
Bruises	Arnica cream or lotion
Sore throat	Throat sprays containing echinacea, thyme oil, licorice, marshmallow, mullein or plantain
Upset tummy	Peppermint oil, ginger lozengers. Fennel tea
Earache	Garlic oil (applied with a cotton wool tip applicator), herbal ear drops containing mullein, skullcap or cohosh root
Toothache	Clove oil or cajeput oil (applied directly to the gums), willow bark tablets
Fevers	Bathe in tepid infusions of yarrow or chamomile. Drink plenty elderflower tea
Sickness & diarrhoea	Artichoke for indigestion, black horehound for nausea & vomiting, strong black tea or charcoal tablets for diarrhoea
Travel sickness	Ginger tablets or sweets

HERBAL FIRST AID (The natural home pharmacy)

General all-purpose remedies:

- **Echinacea** – general all-purpose antimicrobial both internally and externally. It boosts immune responses so good for offering protection against further infection or exacerbation of current infections. Excellent prophylactic to the common cold
- **Tea Tree Oil** – excellent all-round antimicrobial (including fungal infections and protects against parasites eg. lice, ticks, parasitic worms etc…). Very good antiseptic action too so good for preventing further infection but needs to be diluted before use for safety
- **Lavender** – good antiseptic and antimicrobial. Also has pain-relieving properties, it is good for stress & general nervous conditions and it smells nice too! It is one of the few EOs that can be safely use neat.
- **Willow bark tablets** – good all-round painkiller and effective anti-inflammatory

Seek proper advice from a qualified and registered practitioner of herbal medicine on dosages and administration prior to any self-administration.

Specific First Aid

Fever	Elderflower or yarrow tea. Practical measures for cooling the body
Nosebleeds	Cotton wool soaked in witch hazel lotion into nostrils. Practical measures eg. altering head position can help too
Burns & scalds	Aloe vera gel applied directly onto the burn (if you have a fresh plant, cut a fleshy leaf and use the clear, viscous liquid that oozes out from then leaf), marigold tea, witch hazel lotion, green or black tea, plantain or St. John's Wort tea
Fainting	Inhale peppermint oil
Shock	Chamomile , lemon balm or passion flower as a tea
Insect bites & stings	Essential oil of lavender. A good insect repellent is a combination of oils of lavender, citronella, eucalyptus, cedarwood & lemongrass. Limit sugary foods to avoid insects being attracted to the sweet smell released from the body. Also, witch hazel & plantain to apply topically to soothe & heal the skin
Cuts & grazes	Echinacea tincture (topically), tea tree oil & witch hazel cream
Bruises	Arnica, calendula, comfrey & cayenne cream
Sprains & strains Muscle Aches	Arnica, witch hazel & St. John's Wort prepared as a cream or liniment. Oils can be added such as camphor, eucalyptus, rosemary or clove. Comfrey cream (for healing), turmeric tablets (for inflammation)
Splinters	Use flat-ended tweezers to pull out any type of splinter or foreign body in the skin (eg. ticks). Wipe the affected area with tea tree oil, lavender or tincture of echinacea
Allergic reactions	Petasites or butterbur, echinacea, eyebright, chamomile, quercitin supplements
Sunburn	Same as for burns
Preparing dressings	Alginate film dressing is naturally derived from brown seaweed. It forms a gel on contact with a wound to help assist in healing

(iii) Top 20 herbs – a guide to commercial preparations

Administration

There is a vast array of herbal products on the market today both in the UK and in the US, not to mention what can be purchased over the internet. Some manufacturers may place profit and commercial interest over and above ethical considerations and health. This may result in products being made available to the consumer that are of unacceptably poor quality or worse still, pose a health risk due to ingredients being present that have not been verified or checked for safety. Fortunately, both the European and US governments have strict laws to regulate the sale of such herbal medicines but even so, some of the products marketed online continue to challenge the regulators as well as practitioners like me.

Herbs in the US are classified as dietary supplements, not as drugs. This broad category also includes vitamins, minerals, enzymes and other nutritional products. There are many ways in which herbs are marketed and administered, much the same way as conventional drugs. However, commercial brands can vary enormously and product quality is critical in ensuring efficacy of herbal remedies. It is best to get advice from practitioners before purchase.

Preparation type	Comment
Capsules	80% of all herbal supplements are sold in this form. Convenient, palatable & portable. Disadvantage that it contains dried, ground herbs which may lose their potency more quickly. Need to take more of the whole herb extract unlike the concentrated extract. A herbal practitioner could prescribe these and they are taken in a similar manner to conventional medicines ie. before, with or after food.
Teas	Most familiar & traditional form of preparation. Dried leaves and flowers are particularly suited to infusions as it releases important volatile oils (eg. mint, sage, chamomile) but bark, roots, seeds and berries are also used. Usually 2 heaped teaspoons of the dried herb is infused into a cup of boiling water for about 10 minutes. The liquid is strained and drunk at regular intervals depending on the dosage requirements.
Decoctions	Barks, roots, seeds and berries require a little more heat and time to release their medicinal compounds. They need to be simmered on low heat for approx. 10-30 minutes depending on the herb. The liquid is taken at regular intervals depending on the dosage requirements
Tinctures and Glycerites	Fresh or dried herbs are soaked (macerated) in a solvent – alcohol for tinctures and glycerine for gycerites (non-alcoholic) in order to release the active compounds. The process takes a few days and the mixture if filtered to produce the liquid preparation. Concentrations vary

	depending on the herb:solvent ratio ie. Fluid Extract (1:1) being the most concentrated and 1:5 tincture being the least concentrated. Using fresh herbs yield lower concentrations of active constituents than using dried herbs. Usually, a teaspoon of the tincture is taken 3 times a day in a little water before meals but again, this can vary, depending on the dosage requirements.
Standardised Extracts	Preparations that have a known quantity of a key compound or ingredient that is the designated marker of the herb's potency. This gives the assurance of potency & medicinal benefit. Standardised products are available in capsules, tablets & liquid form (tincture or glycerite). There is some argument over the actual benefit of standardisation over whole herb preparations and the synergy of active ingredients.
Tablets	A controlled quantity of finely milled herbal material is compressed and given a thin coating. Some are enteric-coated to prevent stomach acids form altering the active ingredients. These allow absorption of the herb in its original form and concentration in the small intestine without change in its chemical composition. A herbal practitioner may prescribe herbal tablets to be administered in a similar manner to conventional medicines, ie. to be taken at regular intervals before, with or after food.
Infused Oils (fixed oil)	Infused oils are base oils in which herbs have been steeped, usually for several weeks, over low heat or at room temperature eg. St.John's Wort fixed oil or Arnica fixed oil.
Essential Oils (EO)	Essential Oils are chemical concentrations of a plant's volatile oils. Often produced by distillation, EOs are extremely strong and require the supervision of a qualified practitioner before use for medicinal purposes.
Creams, Emollients, Salves & Lotions	Topical preparations (for external use only) which are made in a similar manner to conventional preparations except with the addition of herbs in various forms. Commercial preparations can be good but seek professional advice on brand for product quality and therapeutic effectiveness.

Top 20 Herbs

Herbal supplements and products have become extremely popular in recent years. A wide variety of commercial preparations are now available in most health food shops and supermarkets. Some of the popularly sold herbs are listed here and is by no means comprehensive. The practitioners' list may be entirely different but I have compiled a list of herbs that are commercially popular and have attempted to summarise some of their unique therapeutic properties that makes them special and of great medicinal value to many patients. The herbs have not been listed in any order of priority nor popularity.

Chamomile (*Chamomilla recutita* = German chamomile, *Anthemis nobilis* = Roman chamomile)

Ginkgo (*Ginkgo biloba*)

Echinacea (*Echinacea purpurea*)

Arnica (*Arnica montana*)

Ginger (*Zingiber officinale*)

Garlic (*Allium sativum*)

Artichoke (*Cynara scolymus*)

St.John's Wort (*Hypericum perforatum*)

Chaste berry (*Vitex agnus-castus*)

Valerian (*Valeriana officinalis*)

Devil's claw (*Harpagophytum procumbens*)

Aloe vera (*Aloe barbadensis*)

The ginsengs (*Eleutherococcus senticosis* = Siberian, *Panax ginseng* = Korean, *Withania somnifera* = Indian)

Lavender (*Lavandula angustifolia*)

Tea tree (*Melaleuca alternifolia*)

Mint (*Mentha piperita*)

Marigold (*Calendula officinalis* = pot marigold)

Licorice (*Glycyrrhiza glabra*)

Saw palmetto (*Serenoa repens*)

Cranberry (*Vaccinium macrocarpon*)

1. **Chamomile** is a very popular herb and more so in recent years simply because it is found in many proprietary products as well as commercial teas. It is more commonly sold as a tea, invariably in combination with other herbs that soothe and calm. However, it is also a main ingredient in some herbal creams and lotions because of its excellent anti-inflammatory action. In this respect, it may be useful for skin conditions such as dryness, eczema, allergic reactions which cause redness and swelling etc…Some of the hair products also claim to contain chamomile due to its reputed property of lightening hair colour, particularly light brown hair. It is difficult to comment on this as products will vary and without a proper study into how effective this is, it is really more for cosmetic gain. There are 2 varieties that herbalists use (Roman and German chamomile) and they have slightly differing properties. Both however are anti-inflammatory and antispasmodic so generally quite useful in skin conditions (topical use) and for gut disorders. They are both sedating and relaxing so very useful for stress conditions and symptoms associated with it. Chamomile has the ability to soothe and calm frazzled nerves so anxiety states could benefit enormously from taking this on a regular basis. Taken as a tea is the best for these types of symptoms.

2. **Ginkgo** is another herb that is very popular. It is an excellent circulatory stimulant and can address poor circulation especially to the surface of the skin so cold hands and feet benefit greatly from gingko supplementation. It also improves circulation to the brain and head regions hence its more popular use as an aid to poor memory and brain function. Studies are currently being conducted into its effectiveness in Alzheimer's disease and in other dementia-related disorders. Equally, improving circulation to the head region can help in eyesight problems (eg, macular degeneration and diabetic retinopathy, tinnitus (commonly referred to as 'ringing in the ears'). It is one of the herbs which is commonly sold as a standardised extract, particularly in tablet form. Advice should certainly be sought on commercial brands since it is has a number of known interactions with conventional drugs. Never buy anything from the internet which is not from a reputable source, or without proper professional advice as it should not be taken in certain medical complaints or if you are taking certain medicines as it can produce undesirable, and possibly dangerous interactions.

3. **Echinacea** is one of those herbs that practically everyone has heard of because we have all experienced the common cold. As a prophylactic for the cold and flu, this herb is excellent and some people swear by it for their general immunity and resistance to infection. It is almost too late to start taking it once symptoms appear so it really is best to take it as a supplement if you are susceptible to recurring colds. It is also used topically for minor infections, cuts & grazes (see herbal First Aid) as it is a great antimicrobial and antiseptic. Equally, it is also very good for healing wounds and boosting energy levels in debilitated patients. As a supplement, it is best taken as a standardised extract in capsule or tablet form. For general debility and weakness tinctures are probably better and in combination with other immune boosters, infection-fighting herbs and tonics.

4. **Arnica** is a herb that herbalists only use externally and never on broken skin. Commercial preparations containing arnica are usually designed to treat the symptoms of joint and muscular pain, stiffness or injury and it has excellent healing properties too, particularly for bruises since it encourages blood flow to the skin surface. Oil preparations, lotions or creams are usually combined with other herbs such as rosemary oil, lavender oil or silver birch bark oil and sometimes comfrey base cream. Arnica is also good for rheumatism, varicose veins, sprains, muscular aches and pains.

5. **Ginger** is more renowned for its culinary use than for its medicinal properties but this is rapidly changing. In addition to its wonderful aromatic flavour and distinctive taste, it is an excellent circulatory stimulant, boosting bloodflow to the skin surface. This is particularly useful in conditions associated with poor circulation (eg. chilblains). The more popular use for ginger is really as a tea, especially in digestive complaints such as nausea, vomiting, indigestion and abdominal discomfort. Standardised extracts are best taken for circulatory problems with proper advice beforehand from a medical herbalist because of its known interactions with conventional drugs. It is not suited for patients with 'hot' conditions such as inflammatory disorders because ginger is already a hot herb and will exacerbate the problem.

6. **Garlic** is one of the many herbs where there is proper scientific evidence of its effectiveness. Because of this, many doctors and healthcare practitioners are quite happy to prescribe or recommend garlic as a supplement because of its proven record in a number of medical complaints. Many elderly people prefer to take garlic supplements as opposed to conventional anti-clotting drugs because it also boosts circulation and lowers blood cholesterol. So, as an all-round herb, garlic has more benefits than taking a host of drugs for people who have a number of problems associated with blood disorders. Of course, the fact that it is an excellent antimicrobial agent and can prevent and treat a host of infections is an added bonus. Many of the reputable commercial brands have the necessary required quantities of the active ingredient, which have been made into capsule form and will not degrade easily. Fresh garlic is only effective upon crushing but degrades very easily so must be eaten raw quite quickly to gain any medicinal benefit. This could be a little tricky for one's social life so there is an advantages to taking commercial supplements but it is best to seek proper professional advice from a medical herbalist, particularly on brand and whether there is an existing medical problem or if conventional drugs are already been taken. One of the best things about garlic is that it is big on its antioxidant properties. That is, it has the ability to protect the body against cellular damage often associated with diseases such as cancer and heart disease; very much on the increase in the West.

7. **Artichoke** is fast becoming a very popular supplement, probably because of the growing incidence of heart disease due to high blood cholesterol levels and increased consumption of saturated fats. Interestingly, it has always been popular in Middle-Eastern customs because their diets have traditionally been quite heavy to digest and relatively high in fat. Artichoke is also a very good liver herb in that it protects it against toxins and infections. It also tones & strengthens the liver. It assists digestion and prevents symptoms of poorly digested food. Indirectly it helps in heart disease by lowering blood fats (particularly the triglycerides and cholesterol). It is considered the main herb for the gall bladder.

8. **St. John's Wort** is one of those herbs that has become quite well known for many people. It is taken for depression and anxiety but it also has a host of other important uses. Again, like garlic, there is substantial evidence of its effectiveness in mild to moderate depression (but not for severe depression or psychosis). Many people are familiar with St. John's Wort as a popular and natural alternative to conventional antidepressants. It is often dubbed 'Nature's Prozac'. Though extremely popular as an OTC herbal remedy here in the UK, it is actively prescribed by doctors in Germany in favour of conventional antidepressants for mild to moderate depression. Named after John the Baptist, St. John's Wort contains at least 10 active constituents (AC) that may contribute to its pharmacological effects although herbalists believe that it is the synergy of these ingredients that confers the true therapeutic benefits to the herb. It is effective only in mild to moderate depression, not in severe depression. Its other notable actions are often overlooked since media coverage has largely focused on its antidepressant properties probably because so many people seem to be afflicted with this condition. Importantly, St. John's Wort is effective in combating anxiety and therefore particularly useful in people who experience anxiety along with their depression. It also possesses powerful antiviral properties and is often prescribed for a range of viral infections such as cold sores and the common cold. Topically, it is an excellent vulnerary (wound healer) and an anodyne (pain reliever), prescribed for conditions such as wounds, burns, shingles and musculo-skeletal injury. Medical experts remain undecided as to the clinical usefulness of St. John's Wort despite evidence from rigorous scientific studies and reports of its benefits in many peer-reviewed journals. The list of drug interactions is quite long and varied but includes oral contraceptives, digoxin, anticonvulsants and cyclosporin, amongst others. It is also reported to react dangerously with anti-clotting drug, warfarin, which is commonly prescribed. Side effects may include mild nausea, digestive upset, photosensitivity and fatigue but unlike conventional antidepressants, it does not affect libido or impair the ability to experience orgasm. The recommended daily dose for depression is 900mg of the extract split into 3 doses of 300mg. Herbalists often prescribe St. John's Wort in combination with other herbal nervines as part of an overall treatment plan. Effects can be seen as early as 2 weeks from commencing treatment but it is strongly advisable that a consultation with a qualified and registered practitioner of herbal medicine is sought prior to any self-medication. Empirical science may not value the synergy of the active constituents that lies at the heart of herbal medicine and may

cast doubt on its usefulness in clinical practice. What is clear however is the enormous benefit that it brings to numerous sufferers who simply cannot do without this wonderful herb in a society where depression is such a widespread mental health problem. If taking St. John's Wort is a problem because of possible interactions, consider taking the herb Rhodiola (*Rhodiola rosea*), which is another effective herbal antidepressant with many additional health benefits. Any unwanted side-effects or interactions are yet to be reported for rhodiola.

9. **Chaste berry** is also known as Agnus castus and is considered the main female herb. This is because of its ability to regulate hormones in the female reproductive system. Therefore, it is commonly taken for symptoms associated with problems with this system for eg. PMS (premenstrual syndrome) as part of other measures for balancing the reproductive hormones. In regulating these hormones, some women have successfully addressed a number of problems associated with an abnormal menstrual cycle including infertility, irregular periods, period pain, PMT (premenstrual tension), PCOS (polycystic ovarian syndrome), ovarian cysts and endometriosis (to name a few). Other conditions that would also benefit are acne (for both men and women), heavy menstrual bleeding and conditions of excess oestrogen such as breast cysts and fibroids. It is best taken as a tincture although for convenience, some prefer to take the tablets.

10. **Valerian** is a plant that is found almost world wide and its root has been used medicinally since medieval times. The tincture was widely used in World War I to treat shell shock, including loss of memory and other functions due to prolonged psychological strain. The herb has a pronounced, distinctive odour that is only acquired after harvesting and drying. Valerian's primary traditional use has been as a sedative, namely for the relief of insomnia, anxiety and conditions associated with pain due to muscular cramps. It counteracts nervous tension, excitability, restlessness, stress, panic attacks and irritability. Various clinical trials involving both healthy individuals and patients experiencing poor sleep patterns strongly support the sedating properties of the herb. Studies show that valerian improves quality of sleep without producing the undesirable feelings of 'drowsiness' the following morning that is often associated with conventional sleeping tablets. Standardised extracts should provide a dosage ranging from 150-300mg. This is a single dose that should be taken about half an hour to 45 minutes before bedtime. The dried herb equivalent taken as a tea should provide 1-3g per dose taken at bedtime for insomnia or three times a day for other conditions. Valerian is in general a safe herb even in pregnancy. However, it may cause drowsiness and fatigue in some and it should be avoided altogether if already taking sleeping tablets as it would multiply its effect. Symptoms of overdosing such as headache, nausea, restlessness or visual disturbances can be avoided by following dosage recommendations. In rare instances, it may be stimulating and should never be taken with alcohol. It is strongly recommended that specific advice on dosage and safety is sought from a Medical Herbalist prior to any self-medication.

11. **Devil's Claw** is a popular herbal supplement taken for the pain and discomfort of arthritis. It is also useful for other joint problems too such as gout and tendonitis. It contains important pain-relieving chemicals as well as anti-inflammatories, both characteristics of arthritic conditions. Many patients find that taking regular supplements of this herb improves mobility and lessens the pain, particularly in chronic cases. Many people who enjoy sporting activities and regular physical exercise who are hampered by joint injury or pain, find this a useful supplement in managing their symptoms. Devil's claw also has other benefits including being a digestive stimulant (it is one of the bitterest herbs, taken in tincture form). Traditionally of course, it has been used for centuries by native South Africans to stimulate digestion in addition to controlling pain and fever.

12. **Aloe vera** is a very popular herbal supplement which is taken internally as well as applied externally (topically). It is the juice of the fresh plant that is commonly used and various commercial preparations are sold for a variety of symptoms. Aloe vera gel is the clear viscous liquid that is taken from the inner parts of the long, fleshy leaves. Topically (externally), the gel preparation is commonly used for burns, scalds, minor abrasions, wounds and a variety of skin problems. Taken internally, the gel is said to provide many health benefits and alleviate a number of major disorders such as peptic ulcers, diabetes, cancer, AIDS, inflammatory bowel disease (Crohn's disease and ulcerative colitis) and as a general tonic. However, these claims are yet to be verified through proper, rigorous scientific trials. Commercial preparations of aloe vera gel are available for topical use as well as being a key ingredient in many cosmetic products and toiletries such as skin lotions, creams and moisturisers. The gel is not to be confused with the bitter yellow liquid that is prepared from the outer rind of the leaf. This yellow liquid is often referred to as the sap, latex or aloe juice (or simply aloes) and is quite a strong laxative. Therefore, it is often drunk directly as a digestive aid. Consult a Medical Herbalist about commercial products and brands prior to any self-administration, particularly if it is to be taken internally.

13. **Ginsengs** are medicinal herbs that have been used as tonics for centuries. The 3 main ones that are used within Western herbal medicine are the Siberian ginseng (*Eleutherococcus senticosus*), Asian or Korean ginseng (*Panax ginseng*) and Indian ginseng (*Withania somnifera* also commonly known as Ashwagandha). Despite the similarities in their names, the 3 ginsengs are in fact quite surprisingly, very different to each other and although they share many attributes, notably in their tonic, strengthening and energy boosting properties, they have remarkable differences which make them distinct and unique from each other. All 3 ginsengs are referred to as adaptogens. This means that they enable the body to cope with stress and enable it to adapt to changes that may be potentially damaging to the body. Many people take this herbal supplement for this very reason as they find that they can cope better with the demands of modern life (simply because it is so very stressful) and this enables them to be protected against many of the stress-related illnesses that are common eg,

recurring colds, general fatigue and tiredness, persistent and recurring tension headaches etc….. The great bonus of the ginsengs is that they are also powerful immune stimulants so will boost this system and prevent many of the common infections and illnesses that are often synonymous with feeling 'run-down' and debilitated through prolonged stress. Siberian ginseng is a great female herb though it is not exclusively prescribed for women. It is a tonic herb which has strong immune boosting properties and is a great adaptogen. Women experiencing menopausal symptoms which are accompanied by fatigue and general weakness often find this herb helpful in invigorating them and enabling them to cope with the stressful life change. Tests on the various ginsengs have shown that Siberian ginseng is better for athletic training (increases performance through reducing stress; stress is a known limiting factor in athletic performance). Korean or the Asian ginseng on the other hand has more powerful tonic powers and is regarded more as a 'male' herb simply because of its ability to improve strength and energy levels (a great tonic herb) and boosting immunity (so great for illnesses with general debility). It is also used for convalescence and poor immune function. Ashwagandha or the Indian ginseng is slightly different in character and property to the other ginsengs because it is more sedating and less stimulating than the others so where a more gentle action is required, this is a better choice. Ashwagandha is adaptogenic so is good for stress but unlike the others, it is mildly sedating so if sleep is affected by stress and other symptoms start to appear as a result of poor sleep, this would be my herb of choice. Interestingly it is also good for debility and nervous exhaustion, both common symptoms of prolonged stress. It is also a good immune booster so will combat current infections and confer some protection against any future episodes.

14. **Lavender** is an extremely popular herb and again one that practically everyone would have heard of. Its uses range from scented products and fragrances, to being an ingredient in cosmetics, toiletries and other proprietary products. Its wonderful aroma makes it a highly desirable herb for this very reason. Additionally, lavender has a number of important medicinal benefits and is popularly used in massage oils and rubs in aromatherapy for relieving tension in muscles and to alleviate anxiety. It is quite an effective antispasmodic and therefore relieves muscle spasms that cause tension in these muscles. Lavender is commonly used as an essential oil (EO) and is sedating so used in inhalations, it will be useful in sleep disorders (the oil can be dabbed onto pillows as well to induce sleep). It is also an effective first aid remedy (insect stings/bites and burns). It is also used by herbalists to treat nervous tension to soothe and calm frazzled nerves, plus a range of skin infections such as fungal and bacterial infections including acne (topically). Often it is combined with other EOs into a base oil or cream. Equally, it is added to a herbal cream, lotion or rub for further benefit or simply to make the remedy smell nice. Commercial preparations do vary because of the quality of the herb used for the distillation of the oil. Seek advice first from a herbalist on the brand beforehand especially if it is to be used for medicinal purposes. It is not for internal use unless it is supervised by a health practitioner or herbalist who can prescribe tinctures or teas if it is appropriate.

15. **Tea tree** is a popular herbal remedy as an all round antiseptic and anti-infectious remedy. Topically, it is the EO that is used (diluted in a base oil) for a range of infections caused by a fungus, bacterium, virus or parasite therefore it is usually used to treat conditions such as thrush and athlete's foot (fungal), boils, acne, cystitis (bacterial), herpes (viral) or insect stings/bites plus others. As an ingredient in proprietary products such as shower gels and creams, it is added for its antiseptic properties. It is not for internal use unless under professional guidance and the EO is not to be used neat onto broken skin.

16. **Mint** is a very common culinary herb and has a distinct aroma and flavour. It is popularly drunk as a refreshing tea especially as a digestive aid to ease wind, bloating and indigestion (it is an effective carminative so eliminates trapped air inside the gut). It is a cooling herb so it is popularly added to some toiletries such as shower gels to cool the body down. Topically the EO is often used in sports injuries because of its cooling action (it reduces pain and increases healing). The gel preparations are used for its analgesic properties as it is effective in alleviating pain (eg. nerve pain or headache).

17. **Marigold** is a common garden plant (also known as pot marigold) and popularly marketed as Calendula after its Latin name *Calendula officinalis*. Calendula is renowned for its healing properties, particularly in inflammatory skin conditions such as eczema, minor burns, insect stings and generally for dry skin. Some new brands of cosmetics and toiletries now add calendula to their formulations because of its healing and soothing properties. Topically, calendula is excellent in combating fungal infections eg. vaginal thrush (caused by a yeast-like fungus called *Candida albicans*) although a stronger preparation is usually better for this type of infection. There are a number of effective commercial preparations for use externally, particularly creams, lotions and ointments. For inflamed mucous membranes such as the eyes (eg. conjunctivitis), it combines well with other herbs like witch hazel or eyebright for an effective eye wash. A herbalist should be able to advise on preparation type and administration etc…(as dilution is necessary and dosage considerations are very important). Internally, for the gut, calendula is excellent for peptic ulcers and for other conditions that cause inflammation of the gut lining. Dried leaves can be infused as a tea or used as a gargle for sore throats or any inflammations in the mouth (eg. gingivitis, inflamed gums). It can also be prepared as an infused oil and used topically (externally) for minor injuries or irritations. In Germany, doctors actively use calendula preparations quite readily to heal surgical incisions as well as wounds since marigold is excellent at healing wounds (vulnerary).

18. **Licorice** is a well known plant whose roots have been used for thousands of years in confectionary and flavouring, as well as in herbal medicine, particularly traditional Chinese medicine (TCM). It has

similar uses today in Western herbal medicine because of its strong anti-inflammatory and demulcent properties. Therefore, it is commonly prescribed for conditions such as peptic ulcers, gastritis, and colitis. It is a powerful expectorant and antitussive (prevents coughing) and many commercial preparations include licorice, often in combination with other herbs such as thyme for cough syrups or for other respiratory conditions such as bronchitis or asthma, TB or colds accompanied by a chest infection. Topically, it can be added to creams as it will soothe inflamed membranes, particularly in the gut or mouth (can be used for aphthous ulcers (canker sores). It is also good for a variety of inflammatory skin disorders such as eczema and allergic skin reactions. Licorice is also a hormonal agent and regulates the adrenal gland which secretes adrenaline and oestrogen (amongst other hormones) so it can be prescribed for hormone-related and stress-related conditions such as the menopause and symptoms associated with it. The sweet taste of licorice makes it an ideal herb for preparations that are very bitter and is particularly appealing to children. However, it should not be taken by patients who have high blood pressure as it will make it worse.

19. **Saw palmetto** is viewed favourably by many doctors and other conventional healthcare practitioners as an effective anti-inflammatory in benign prostatic hyperplasia (BPH). BPH which can progress onto prostate cancer is on the increase and many men seek to find herbal treatments for the symptoms rather than consider surgery or long-term drug therapy. Much of the need for invasive surgery in the growing incidence of BPH can be eliminated with the use of saw palmetto extract which appears to offer greater appeal to both patients and doctors because there is adequate scientific evidence to prove its effectiveness. In the US, it has been found to be the sixth best-selling herb whilst extracts of saw palmetto berry are being used extensively throughout the world for the relief of BPH. Both the French and German governments approve the herbal extracts for this purpose. Positive results with saw palmetto have been confirmed in numerous open as well as double-blind, placebo-controlled clinical trials. All of these studies demonstrate statistically significant improvements in the symptoms of BPH, which include increased volume and rate of urine flow, alleviation of pain, night time urinations and decreased numbers of voidings per day. Overall, these studies showed a consistent benefit of saw palmetto extract with virtually no side effects of any consequence. Recommendations of dietary measures in conjunction with this herb, in particular supplementations of selenium and zinc show remarkable improvements in symptoms. Most patients who take this supplement experienced relief within days of beginning the therapy, with benefits continuing to improve over time in many cases, as much as one year of continuing improvement. Saw palmetto is relatively safe to use long-term with no serious side effects being officially recorded. Moreover, the safety profile of this herbal preparation is very good, appealing to those who are concerned about toxicity issues and potential complications, as well as to those currently on conventional drugs for other conditions that are symptomatic of age and decline. Though the commercial preparations are used mainly for BHP, this herb is very much a tonic herb and a hormonal agent. It can sometimes be prescribed for impotence or male sterility and general debility.

20. **Cranberry** is in the same family as blueberry and bilberry and shares some of their wonderful antioxidant properties. However, its reputed action is really in preventing urinary tract infections (UTIs). It is a well tolerated and safe herbal remedy and it has great anti-infective properties especially in those susceptible to UTIs. There is some scientific evidence to support its medicinal benefits and because of this many doctors and healthcare practitioners are happy to endorse the taking of this herbal supplement rather than prescribing repeated doses of conventional antibiotic treatment in a range of urinary tract disorders and infections. Commercial preparations are readily available as tablets but it is strongly recommended that proper advice is sought on brand prior to purchase.

Self-Administration

With the increasing popularity and availability of herbal products, especially via the internet, it becomes ever more pressing to educate and inform on the dangers of indiscriminate self-administration. By far the most problematic is the issue of herb-drug interactions as many patients are unaware that taking herbal supplements whilst on conventional drugs could have potential adverse reactions. Equally, doctors and health care practitioners need to be aware of these dangers and whilst literature on the subject is not exhaustive, there is information on the dangers of widely prescribed drugs along with self-administration of herbal supplements. Additionally, not all patients are informed about contra-indications and may self-administer without realising the dangers of taking herbal supplements when they have an existing medical condition or disorder. Many people think that all herbs are safe because it is a natural product and think that it will be harmless at any dose. This is not always the case and there is a danger of overdosing. Herbal products should be viewed in the same manner as any conventional drug giving due regard to side effects, maximum dosage and contra-indications. Proper, informative advice should always be sought before considering any herbal treatment, however minor the ailment or condition.

(iv) The role of the Herbal Medicine Practitioner

What is a herbal medicine practitioner?

A Western herbal medicine practitioner is an alternative health practitioner who has been trained like conventional doctors in making a diagnosis and in case-history taking. Instead of prescribing drugs however, a herbalist will prescribe a course of herbal medicines. The emphasis here is on treating the person rather than just treating the symptoms. The symptoms are viewed in light of other factors so diagnosis and treatment is therefore very much within a holistic context. Herbal treatments can vary from recommending simple dietary and lifestyle changes to prescribing herbal remedies over a course of weeks or months depending on the severity of the problem or how chronic it is.

Why you should consult a herbalist

Herbal medicines are effective medicines when used appropriately and correctly. Many people are unclear about the many different remedies, particularly the vast array of commercial brands and product types or formulations on the market today. Herbal medicines work on all types of conditions and ailments but its potency and therapeutic abilities are best highlighted in chronic or long-standing conditions especially those that have not responded to conventional treatments. This may be due to a number of factors but one reason could be that the condition being treated has more underlying causes that only a holistic form of treatment will address. Regarding symptoms in isolation is rather like placing a sticking plaster to a problem that has more fundamental causes in origin and offers only a temporary solution. This becomes more evident in light of recent and important findings in the mind-body link or psychoneuroimmunology (PNI). A herbalist will consider the symptoms as part of a whole (exploring the mind as well as the body) and make recommendations that actively involve the patient in the decisions for treatment and any changes to lifestyle or diet.

Importantly, herbalists have been trained to choose the most appropriate herb(s) for the condition being treated, in addition to how to administer and type of preparation that is suitable for the patient with dosage and safety considerations. It is not a case of one treatment fits all, more a case of tailor-making a formula to suit the individual patient. It is always advisable to consult a qualified and registered practitioner of herbal medicine rather than taking endless quantities of herbal supplements (which may or may not be appropriate or indeed of good quality). Worse still, indiscriminately taking any number of herbal remedies based on a single report (probably taken out of context) or a finding or favourable press article can lead to all sorts of problems and complications in symptoms with new ones emerging and limiting the progress of treatment of the original problem. Remember, medical herbalists are highly trained practitioners who will be able to give you a better understanding of your symptoms and treat you in the context of all outside factors in your life. What is more, they will prescribe the most appropriate herbal remedies for you that is tailor-made for you only using medicines that are of high quality at dosages that are effective and safe.

Training requirements for a herbalist – what does a qualified, registered practitioner mean?

In the past, training requirements have varied and could have ranged from a matter of weeks to a matter of years. However, recent changes in European legislation has attempted to regulate this training process as well as the practice of herbal medicine to make it more consistent and to ensure that all herbalists have undergone the same training and practise in the same way, wherever you live in Europe. Importantly, this is to ensure public safety, particularly as herbal medicines are potent chemicals but also to give due importance and recognition to the profession of herbal medicine. Discussions are still in progress on how to proceed with implementing such changes but until such time that matters are finalised, it remains the priority of the individual professional bodies to regulate their members in how they practise and to stipulate certain requirements before being accepted as a member. Part of this involves the training process.

A fully qualified medical herbalist has undergone an extensive training programme (quite often a degree programme) that includes a substantial amount of clinical training. This can be a number of years. Clinical training is where the theory is put into practice (very much like the training for conventional doctors) and students who see patients are supervised by an experienced herbal practitioner and clinician. Tests and examinations have to be passed at various stages of the training programme before a student can proceed to ensure that an accredited institution passes practitioners that are competent, fully qualified and have the ability to practise safely. Moreover, the final stages of training require that students satisfy test criteria and assessments overseen by conventional doctors and other medical practitioners.

Most practitioners are registered with a professional body that regulates their practice and often assigns an experienced Mentor in their first few years of clinical practice. Members of a recognised professional body invariably have letters after their name to indicate which professional body or association that they are a part of eg. MNIMH being a Member of the National Institute of Medical Herbalists, MCPP being a Member of the College of Practitioners of Phytotherapy or MBHMA being Member of the British Herbal Medicine Association. Equally, in America, there is the American Herbalist Guild (AHG) or Naturopathic Doctor or ND which implies that they have had training as a naturopathic doctor. NDs are conversant in natural approaches to healthcare and treatment which includes herbal medicines and nutrition.

However, just because a herbalist does not have the prerequisite letters after their name does not mean that they cannot help you. It may have been that their knowledge and expertise has been acquired through tradition. They may be self-taught, or gained information that has been passed on through generations of their ancestors. Perhaps there were no specific training or educational programmes available at that time. It is important not to dismiss them simply because they do not have the necessary letters after their names. They may have much wisdom and experience in the application of herbs that no educational training programmes can teach. Remember that even some of these training programmes and qualifications have no legal status beyond the completion of that course of study. One of the best and reliable ways to ensure you get a reputable and credible practitioner is through referrals, either from other complementary and alternative healthcare practitioners, doctors or therapists within mainstream medicine. Don't be afraid to ask awkward questions, from cost to their claims!

When you should consult a herbalist

It is never too late or indeed too early to consult a medical herbalist. They are trained to refer in cases which are serious and where conventional intervention is necessary. It is never too early as simple changes to lifestyle and diet may be adequate to address the current problem. Herbalists are trained in the same diagnostic skills as conventional doctors so the time to seek advice would be as soon as symptoms appear or when you feel unwell, even though there are no symptoms. In moments like these, never underestimate your own perception of feeling unwell. It may become necessary to inform your doctor or healthcare practitioner that you are consulting a herbalist as this will need to be taken into consideration when reviewing your symptoms and to share critical information.

What to expect from a consultation

Medical herbalists are trained in the same way as conventional doctors regarding diagnosis. The first consultation involves the taking of a case history which examines the presenting complaint, symptoms, the past medical history, the family history and a systematic enquiry. In the holistic context, the family and social history is considered in addition to a thorough review of diet and lifestyle. Sometimes a physical examination may be necessary in order to make or confirm a diagnosis. Follow up consultations are usually shorter and will monitor the progress of the treatment.

CHAPTER 4 – HERBAL HEALING

(i) Tonic herbs and optimising health

'Prevention is better than cure'. To some, this phrase epitomises their fundamental beliefs and constitutes an essential health philosophy that is integral to their lives. As lifestyles become increasingly hectic, with daily routines dominated by demanding schedules, the impracticalities of adopting healthier lifestyles are defined by these constraints. The decline in natural body processes that accompany the physical aspects of age dictates that preventing illness is not always possible in the current climate of stress, heavy professional workloads and personal commitments. Moreover, combined with the increasing virulent nature of some of the diseases witnessed today, it is undoubtedly the case that the pattern of disease and prevalence will be indicative of these changes within our society.

It is an inevitable course of nature that we will fall ill at some point during our life. The human body is a remarkable natural machine, not only in design but also in its performance and recovery abilities. It can carry out an extraordinary number of functions with precision, accuracy and timing, conserving energy all the while. Its capacity for repair, regeneration and adaptation following injury or stress is to be marvelled considering the perpetual strain the body is put under. To appreciate the full extent of our inherent physiological mechanisms that keep our systems in proper working order, is to recognise and value the episodes in which the body remains disease-free rather than focus entirely on the duration and frequency in which the body becomes susceptible to infection and disease.

The reference to disease is not as life-threatening as it implies. It is more a case of minor ailments and injuries that plague most of us from time to time. However, the majority of the common complaints can be avoided by implementing a number of precautionary measures such as ensuring a well balanced diet, taking adequate exercise, limiting alcohol intake, avoiding smoking etc.… Recent concerns surrounding health issues such as the potential health risks of the MMR vaccine, HRT and OTC (over the counter) cholesterol-reducing drugs such as statins, now being debated over whether it should be included in our drinking water further reinforces the importance of natural approaches to optimising good health.

The gentle action of herbs (as described in Chapter 2) means that they can be easily incorporated into daily routines to improve and enhance good health. Overall health and well-being can be significantly improved through cleansing the system and eliminating toxins. The tonic actions of some of the more selective herbs that exert a stronger and more specific action is just as important. Moreover, herbs that boost immune responses and defence mechanisms in the body are equally important in preventing illness or a recurrence of infections that are organic in origin. The focus of any optimisation should reflect the detoxifying action of the liver, bowel, skin and kidneys in addition to the blood circulation and lymphatic drainage. Over time and combined with supplementary health strategies, achieving an enhanced state of health, both physically and mentally will have a dramatic effect on improving the overall quality of life.

Much of what is discussed here is very much in context with our changing attitudes to health as well as the practical considerations which dictate the decisions over dietary and lifestyle modifications. Socio-economic factors and environmental influences have an equal impact, in addition to our perception of body image and the concept of what is regarded as 'healthy'. Further, genetic predisposition (susceptibility or risk) cannot be discounted but neither should it dominate any overriding concerns about health since environmental influences (such as lifestyle changes) have shown to significantly influence health and well-being despite an established risk. Optimum health and incorporating herbs should be viewed in its entirety taking into account such factors whether it is to improve current health status or to treat and manage a specific medical complaint.

As described in previous chapters, the herbal approach to preventing illness involves the use of herbs that assist the body in maintaining balance in all physiological systems. This essentially involves eliminating and cleansing the body of toxins, preventing toxic build up, strengthening, toning and supporting major organs and systems. Targeting the immune system directly could also be beneficial in those who are prone to infection especially those under persistent stress, those whose nutritional intake is of poor quality, those who do not sleep well or those who have variable sleep patterns like shift work.

Equally, the blood and lymph circulations are crucial in providing adequate defence in combating infection and disease. Optimising health has to address this is just as important as tackling the key organs and systems of detoxification and elimination. In some cases, specific organs can be targeted such as a sluggish liver, poor gut function leading to poor absorption of essential nutrients and poor elimination of waste products. The following organs and systems are all involved in optimising health:

1. Liver   detoxification & elimination
2. Bowel   digestion, assimilation & elimination
3. Kidneys   elimination
4. Skin   elimination & defence
5. Lungs   elimination & defence
6. Blood circulation   defence & elimination
7. Lymphatic circulation   defence & elimination
8. Immune system   defence

1. Liver

The liver is one of the most important organs within our body and yet poorly emphasised and looked after. It performs over 500 functions and is one of the largest organs in our body. Its capacity for repair and regeneration is phenomenal considering the enormous demands placed upon it, in addition to the stress it faces with our poor diets and lifestyle practices. The liver is among the few internal human organs capable of natural regeneration of lost tissue; as little as 25% of remaining liver can regenerate into a whole liver again.

One of the crucial aspects of liver function is its role in detoxification. The basic principle of this has been explained in the earlier chapters. Popularly termed 'detox', the liver is instrumental in ensuring that all toxins and potentially harmful products of metabolism are rendered safe in order that the body can eliminate them before they accumulate within the blood and tissues. Ensuring that this happens effectively, requires an efficient circulatory system which will transport the toxic chemicals to the appropriate organs of elimination.

To discuss the true importance of the liver is beyond the scope of this book. Suffice it to say however, that many of the common complaints and conditions such as fat intolerance, poor digestion, bloating, weight fluctuations, IBS etc… can be attributed to the poor functioning of the liver. Many of us are unaware of the extent of our liver damage and have probably got accustomed to its substandard functioning. Herbal detox programmes are becoming very popular as the real importance of the liver becomes fully recognised and respected.

The liver is also involved in bile production. Bile is an important digestive substance that assists fat digestion and helps keep the acid-base balance of the gut environment so that the enzymes can work. Many of the problems associated with fat intolerance are mainly due to poor bile production from the liver. A congested and over-burdened liver cannot function efficiently and must be addressed as part of any treatment plan, particularly in the elderly where digestive problems can be acute owing to the decline in digestive function with age. There are a number of herbs that can address poor liver functioning which will indirectly improve digestive function as a result.

Notable liver herbs have a broad action on the organ, assisting, supporting, toning, strengthening and even protecting it. These herbs are described generally as hepatics and hepatoprotectives. Equally, some herbs directly improve bile production by the liver or its release from the gall bladder where it is stored. Other herbs can influence the regeneration process thereby improving its efficiency and functioning. Some liver herbs are directly involved in the biochemical detoxification pathways that render toxic chemicals and by-products of metabolism less harmful and suitably safe for elimination.

Good examples of liver herbs:

Dandelion (*Taraxacum officinale*)   - mild laxative (root)
                                         - diuretic

	- ↑ appetite (bitter herb) - ↑ bile production & secretion
Milk Thistle (*Silybum marianum*)	- protects liver cells from damage - ↑ repair & regeneration of liver cells
Artichoke (*Cynara scolymus*)	- protects liver cells - ↑ appetite (via bitter action) - ↑ bile production - a general liver tonic
Chinese magnolia vine (Schisandra) (*Schisandra chinensis*)	- protects liver against damage - has detoxification properties
Fumitory (*Fumaria officinalis*)	- normalises bile production & secretion
Turmeric (*Curcuma longa*)	- improves detox role of liver - ↑ bile production
Barberry (*Berberis vulgaris*)	- ↑ bile production - improves poor liver function - improves poor gut function (indirectly)

Aspects of herbal detox and fasting

A consequence of modern living and a Western lifestyle places an unnatural burden on the liver. Herbal detox programmes currently in favour with many celebrities are essentially based on cleansing the system of the chemical and metabolic debris that have accumulated over the years. This is partly achieved by boosting the synergistic action of the digestive system and the liver, which both assist in eliminating the toxins from reaching our tissues. Poor digestive function and liver performance will impact greatly on the body's ability to limit toxic overload and its accumulation in our cells. The purpose of detox therefore is to remove these unwanted debris and toxins that have been stored up over time in order to cleanse the body and revive flagging organs that have been overworked.

Most detox programmes will involve some aspect of boosting liver performance and digestive function in its elimination of waste material. A poorly performing liver will not detoxify substances effectively and there is a danger of toxic load to the cells. Similarly, a congested gut will reabsorb waste into the cells via the bloodstream which will undoubtedly have health consequences later on. In improving matters, a herbalist may prescribe liver detox herbs such as turmeric or schisandra. To protect the liver from further damage, milk thistle may also be prescribed. Importantly, some vegetables such as the brassicas (eg. Broccoli,

Brussels sprouts, cabbage, horse radish etc..) also contain key enzymes that have been shown to possess certain cancer-preventing properties in addition to boosting liver detox activity.

Digestive tonics, laxatives and liver tonics are important components of any herbal detox programme. The health and function of the colon (large part of the lower gut where most of the waste is determined) is just as important in general health, particularly if symptoms such as bloating, abdominal distension/discomfort, IBS symptoms, constipation etc… are to be avoided. However, fasting is another way in which the body can eliminate stored toxins from tissues by providing the necessary respite to essential organs such as the liver and bowels. This gives these vital systems the chance to rest, recuperate and repair and will certainly provide a welcome relief from the continual demands placed on them. There are of course various types of fasting and should be chosen according to constitution, the individual, personality and in my view, with proper supervision to assess any medical risk associated with this kind of regime and if effective results are to be seen.

Fruit-only, vegetable-only or water-only fasts are just a few of the many types that are advised. The aim of any fast is essentially to encourage the release of stored toxins from cells and tissues into the bloodstream. Once in the bloodstream, they are then likely to be taken to the kidneys to be eliminated from the body. Releasing toxins from the cells has many benefits from improving energy levels, improving the functioning of vital organs, improving the clarity and quality of the skin and surrounding tissues, improving mental clarity, eliminating symptoms such as fatigue, lethargy, persistent headaches, joint pains and muscular aches to name a few. Importantly, fasting also eases congestion and burden on important detoxification organs and systems such as the liver and gut.

Most advocates of fasting will only really advise it for short periods followed by changes to an existing diet or regimen that is poor in nutritional value. The general discomfort and sickness often initially experienced by those who attempt fasting is an indication of the extent of toxin release in to the bloodstream. Circulating toxins cause the side-effects often seen such as nausea, headache, malaise, stomach cramps, general fatigue and weakness. For this reason, it is not advisable to continue on a fasting 'diet' for any longer than for 2 consecutive days at any given time as it may do more harm than good. Remember, the kidneys and the circulatory system will have to excrete these products and they don't need to face a sudden onslaught of these toxins which may be more than the organs can cope with. Fasting should always be supported by proper nutritional and medical advice.

The benefits of fasting is a contentious issue within conventional science and medical circles. However, if carried out safely and sensibly with proper nutritional advice, perhaps assisted by herbal support, the many benefits experienced by those who fast will far outweigh the critical evidence of poorly planned and executed programmes. It is important to note that some of the major religions in the world incorporate fasting into their daily lives and cultural practices. In certain traditions, it is often closely associated with a spiritual and religious basis for its practice combined with the emphasis on mind, body and spirit.

FOODS THAT ARE GOOD FOR THE LIVER	
Vegetables	**Fruits**
The brassicas (cabbage, Brussels sprouts, broccoli, horse radish)	Apples
Artichoke (both globe & Jerusalem)	Grapefruit
Beetroot	Grapes
Alfalfa sprouts	Lemons
Herbs & spices (eg. garlic, fennel, parsley, onions)	Pears
Watercress	Apricots
	Avocado
	Pineapple & Papaya
	Watermelon

2. Bowel

Colon health is an important issue but it is not just this part of the digestive system that is important. Good nutrition and a healthy lifestyle will optimise the health of the entire system and ensure good digestion all round. Of particular importance in detox is the function of the colon, part of the lower gut. This part of the bowel is responsible for the absorption of water and additional nutrients that were also absorbed in the earlier sections of the gut. Optimum functioning of this system ensures that an adequate balance of ions, nutrients, water, pH etc…is maintained to continue the biochemical reactions, fluid levels (hydration), electrolyte balance, acid-alkaline balance (pH) etc…Importantly, proper removal of waste will ensure that the system does not get clogged up with toxins and worse still, to get reabsorbed back into the blood stream to circulate into various other systems. This will undoubtedly exacerbate any existing illness and almost certainly be the cause of others commonly seen eg. arthritis, headaches, sleep disorders and many more. This portion of the gut is also where waste material is formed because most of the water is absorbed in this region of the gut.

Most people suffer from constipation because of poor dietary habits. This can be remedied in two ways: herbal laxatives (which may work by increasing gut motility and stimulate the gut muscles to push material through the gut) or through bulk laxatives which provide sufficient fibre/bulk for stool formation so that the muscles do not strain in eliminating any waste (straining contributes to haemorrhoids or piles, a common disorder which can be easily remedied). In the short term, herbal laxatives can be very useful in kick starting a sluggish system and giving the system a good clear out. Any lingering toxic waste material can be removed in this way. However, I do not advocate laxatives for any longer periods of time and certainly not as a mainstay for any herbal lifestyle choice. Long-term use of laxatives (herbal or conventional) can make the system very lazy and the muscles responsible for eliminating waste from the lower part of the gut can become highly dependent on laxatives. Cramping and spasms of these muscles can also occur with inappropriate use of laxatives and does not encourage the system to work by itself in eliminating waste material from the body. The long-term strategy for any change is to ensure that the system can work on its own and work to its optimum capacity. My advice is usually to use gentle laxatives, although in cases where stronger action is required, I will prescribe it for a short period only. Examples of herbal laxatives have been mentioned in earlier chapters. Following this, I recommend effective dietary changes that patients can realistically adhere to and to incorporate these changes into their life so that it can be maintained on a long-term basis and through proper nutritional changes without a dependency on laxatives. The later sections on nutrition will provide some advice and recommendations on effective dietary changes and in improving gut health the natural way. This is the only effective long-term solution to any digestive disorders and in optimising bowel function.

3. Kidneys

The kidneys are important elimination organs and given little attention by most of us, until something goes wrong. Flushing out the blood of impurities and metabolic waste from the liver and digestive system requires hard work including a good diet based on drinking plenty of water. To really fully appreciate the efficient functioning of the kidneys, one has to have experienced kidney infection or damage. Their capacity for clearing the blood of toxins and maintaining the delicate balance of important chemicals such as electrolytes, ions and the pH balance is phenomenal considering the burden they are faced with on a daily basis. Optimising the health of the kidneys can be easily achieved through proper, sustained dietary and lifestyle practices that include drinking plenty of water and a balance of nutrients. Fluid intake is particularly important, especially plain water because it assists the kidneys in providing the medium in which to flush out toxins and to dilute their harmful effects. In simple terms, the more water that is drunk, the easier it is for the kidneys to prevent toxic build up or for them to concentrate to any significant level. It also prevents any infection setting in due to the dilution effect and the mechanical effect of the kidney flushing out any infective agent from its system.

A lack of water has the effect of concentrating the toxins and debris in the blood so increasing the risk of infection and general malaise. The kidneys are particularly susceptible to infection due to lack of water as it is here that the blood is filtered and waste is eliminated. Herbs that are traditionally used for improving kidney function usually exert a diuretic effect thus supporting the detox activity of the liver and bowel. Herbal diuretics such as dandelion, nettle and celery are all excellent choices in this regard. Equally, natural anti-infective agents such as cranberries (as juice) or ripe juniper berries (as tincture or tea) are good choices especially if the system is susceptible to kidney or bladder infections. Juniper berries is my herb of choice in cases where there are symptoms of rheumatic conditions (eg. gout, arthritis) in addition to urinary tract infections.

Toxic build up in tissues, cells and blood present a number of problems, notably in damage and destruction of important anatomical structures but also in triggering inflammatory responses. This is because the body recognises such toxins as foreign material and recruits the inherent mechanisms of our immune defence system to do whatever it can to limit the attack. Therefore, improving the function of our organs of elimination becomes vital particularly if there are existing inflammatory conditions, such as acne or arthritis for example. Both of these conditions benefit enormously from detoxification and elimination.

4. Skin

The skin is the largest organ in the body. Hard to imagine this as an 'organ' as such, but it is and carries out the essential functions of elimination and defence. It acts as a mechanical barrier to the outside world, protecting the body and its delicate organs and tissues from the harsh environment, whilst enabling it to interact very closely with it in terms of gaining important nutrients for gaseous exchange. You can tell a lot by a person's skin, from their facial complexion to levels of hydration, skin tone, elasticity, suppleness and shine. The general appearance of the skin is almost always a good indicator of the state of health, nutritional status and effects of stress.

The skin is regarded as an organ of elimination because of the process of sweating, which removes toxins, impurities, metabolic waste and water. Sweating also serves an important purpose in temperature regulation because the mere evaporation of sweat from the body requires heat. Of course, seasonal changes dictate that levels of sweating decrease significantly in winter months. This is why regular exercise is so important in order to continue the elimination function of the skin, in addition to gaining the host of other benefits that exercise provides.

To make the skin efficient at elimination, it is important to feed it properly and therefore nutrition is foremost, a priority. Adequate exercise is equally important in order to ensure good blood flow to the skin surface. Toxins to be removed will be in the blood so it is important to bring them to the surface so that they can be eliminated effectively from the sweat pores. Good skin health also involves physical and manual techniques such as exfoliation, skin brushing and massage. All will benefit the skin by removing dead skin cells from the outer layer (epidermis) and so prevent it from clogging up the pores and improving its appearance on the whole. Fundamentally, a good cleansing routine that is compatible with skin type is absolutely necessary as this will remove dirt and impurities from getting embedded in the skin, clogging up the pores and at worst, causing infection or inflammation. Poor cleansing or a lack of it will almost certainly prevent the skin from breathing, leading to its lacklustre appearance, spots & pimples, dryness, irritation and recurrent skin infections. But of course, all of these practical measures are of little consequence if the nutrition is poor and the lifestyle is less than adequate. The basics of skin health are described in more detail in Chapter 5 (Health Essentials)

5. Lungs

The lungs, like the digestive tract, can be considered to be our internal skin and considerably expansive in surface area to perform an important elimination function. Removal of respiratory waste, in particular carbon dioxide (CO_2), ensures that this waste material does not accumulate in the blood. Poor lung function not only deprives cells and tissues of the all important oxygen (O_2), but causes an imbalance of the ratio between the two gases. Rising levels of CO_2 in the blood upsets the delicate acid-alkaline balance in our systems. This can lead to all sorts of problems in biochemical reactions resulting in metabolic disturbances that trigger a host of illnesses.

Improving lung function has many benefits, not least of which is efficient oxygen delivery to cells and tissues, maintenance of the correct acid-alkaline balance in our system. Of course, we all know that smoking is detrimental to lung health but equally, so is poor air quality. Current concerns on climate change, globalisation and pollution effects are justified since we have little control over the air we breathe, particularly in large cities. However, I always advise my patients to spend as much time as is feasible in the countryside, where there is a greater chance of better air quality. This often reminds me of the time when doctors and physicians in previous centuries used to actively prescribe a stint to the seaside or the country as part of the treatment plan for their patients. Now of course, one can easily see the wisdom of this advice only too readily in light of increasing incidence of asthma, allergies, respiratory disorders and a host of other illnesses due to environmental effects. Damage to the breathing apparatus is not only caused by cigarette smoking but also by air pollution and the lungs have to work even harder at obtaining the O_2 from the air and delivering it to the blood for transport to cells and tissues.

6. Blood circulation

The blood has many functions. Its role in optimum health is really in defence and elimination. Poor circulation is never a health benefit. It is difficult to understand why some people have a very good circulation and why others don't. One thing is pretty certain, circulation always declines with age, as with many other processes combined with anatomical changes. However, herbal tonics usually address some aspect of circulation, either centrally (heart, lungs, gut) or to the surface of the body (blood vessels to or near the skin surface). Both types of circulatory stimulants are vital because everything that the body does and our mere existence depends very much on a proper, efficient and effective circulation.

In its capacity of defence, the blood is responsible for transporting important antibodies and agents of our immune systems to the site of infection, damage or general defence. Circulating antibodies serve as a reminder of past infection but there are mechanisms on standby should the body be under attack at any time. If blood circulation was deficient in any way, the defence system of the body is very much compromised. Recurring illness is often a sign of a poor circulatory system and depending on the condition being treated, circulatory stimulants serve a very important purpose in boosting recovery. Herbs that are generally prescribed for addressing circulation, either centrally, locally or for general health of the blood vessels transporting the blood, are hawthorn, bilberry, ginkgo, garlic or ginger.

The blood circulatory system also has a crucial role in elimination in that it transports waste products and unwanted metabolites to the relevant organs of elimination (notably the kidneys, skin and lungs here). Without an effective transport system, toxic build up occurs and a redistribution of these waste materials into other parts of the body. Further, the accumulation of such toxins and waste cause damage and can limit the effective workings of a particular organ or system. Illness is very much a sign of such disturbances and poor elimination of such waste material. Blood circulation is always considered alongside any treatment rationale as it is vital to the treatment process.

7. Lymphatic circulation

The lymphatic system is another circulatory system, though given little regard for the important work that it does. Primarily, it is part of our immune system as well as transporting nutrients (like then blood) to various parts of the body. Its circulation should be viewed in the same manner as the blood because any sluggishness in lymph fluid circulation has implications on health and well-being. Just like the blood circulation, it is important for the lymphatic circulation to work effectively. The circulating fluid is called lymph and it surrounds every cell in our body and acts as a intermediary between the blood and the cells. It is a two-way circulation that connects tissues and cells with the blood circulation. It is responsible for transporting waste substances from the cells that are filtered by the lymph nodes and spleen. Lymph vessels connect up with the blood at other sites in the body is also an important part of our defence system in that it contains specialised cells of immunity. The lymph glands (located in specific areas of the body) contain important immune cells that constantly work to filter the lymph of toxins but also to ensure immunity from harmful or infectious agents. You may notice that in times of illness, infection or a serious illness, the lymph nodes (commonly referred to as 'glands') are usually swollen. This can signify a number of things but in the most common cases, it due to infection and an indication that the defence cells have multiplied to improve their attack on the infectious agent.

A poorly functioning lymphatic system can lead to many disorders due to it being over-burdened with toxins, poor lymphatic drainage and swollen glands. Formation of cellulite is commonly attributed to the build up of toxins due to poor drainage from the lymphatic system, not assisted by diet, lifestyle or the manner in which it is laid down under the skin. Toxic build up is an ideal breeding ground for chronic conditions such as arthritis, skin conditions such as acne and glandular disorders (to name but a few). The herbal approach to tackling this problem is essentially to restore a free flowing lymphatic system and to clear the toxic overload. In this regard, depurtives (alteratives) are vital to the treatment rationale as are immune agents to ensure that any lingering infection is dealt with before the system can be totally free from invasion. Effective depuratives are cleavers, red clover, blue flag or poke root (amongst others). Good immune agents are goldenseal, echinacea, astragalus or ginseng. Marigold (calendula) is a general all-round herb for the lymphatic system Again, depending on the condition being treated and on the patient profile, the herbal prescription will vary. Some gain great benefit also from manipulation techniques as an addition to the herbal treatment. A specific type of massage called lymphatic drainage focuses on key areas of the body where the massage movements go in the direction of the lymph circulation thus encouraging, enhancing and improving lymph circulation and ultimately its drainage. This in turn will encourage the elimination of toxins due to its release from the lymphatic system into the blood stream for removal from the body.

Other measures such as dietary changes should include an avoidance of strong foods, particularly highly fatty foods and high protein foods as these are not easy to digest and can take its toll on an already exhausted system. So, temporarily cut out or limit the following:

- Fried foods
- Red meats (replace with white meats and fish)
- Sugar and foods high in sugar especially refined sugar
- Dairy products eg. high fat cheese, milk, butter, cream, lard, suet
- Alcohol
- Pre-packed foods and ready meals
- Foods high in artificial substances eg. hydrogenated fats/ trans fatty acids
- Foods high in hydrogenated fats & trans fatty acids eg. cakes, biscuits, chocolates

Replacing some or all of the above foods with a high proportion of fruit, vegetables and water will not only give the lymphatic system a chance to recover but will also act to cleanse the system by eliminating the backlog of toxins that have accumulated over time. For a proper assessment of the toxic burden and how to address this safely it is best to consult a herbal medicine practitioner who can work out a phased programme of sensible diet and lifestyle changes and herbal treatments that are specific to ensure the optimum health of the lymphatic system.

8. Immune System

We have all heard of being 'run down' and often associate that with our immune system and a reduced ability to fight off infection. There is ample observational evidence to suggest the negative impact of stress on the immune system as seen by recurring infection and illness, fatigue, lethargy or general malaise. However, to establish a link between stress and reduced immunity through proper scientific study has been more difficult to prove. In keeping in line with holistic care, it is important to look beyond identifying and eradicating the infectious agent. Examining other factors such as the environment, stress effects, the emotional and psychological status of the patient as contributory factors should also be given due regard. For many, there is invariably some aspect of stress that features in the infective state.

The main purpose of the immune system is in defence. There are many components such as antibodies, blood cells and lymph nodes as well as organs such as the spleen and liver. In any health programme involving optimum health, it is important to address immune function and the manner and extent to which the defence mechanisms of the body are working. After addressing obvious target areas such as stress management, lifestyle changes, diet and environmental triggers, herbal supplements can be used to boost a flagging immune system and to prevent infection. Common immune boosters include echinacea, ginseng, goldenseal and garlic. A herbalist will be able to choose the most appropriate herb, dosage and the combination in any herbal prescription for each patient. It is important to note that there is little value in taking herbal supplements to boost immunity if it is not in conjunction with other measures such as nutritional changes, lifestyle modifications and the effective management of stress.

(ii) Herbal alternatives for common ailments (A-Z)

Many of us suffer from recurring problems and conditions that are common. Some are potentially serious, some are on the increase whereas others are a real nuisance and difficult to eradicate. The following section attempts to explain the origins of these common problems and disorders, as well as the reasoning behind the herbal treatment or management of those conditions. It is by no means detailed in its explanation and the remit of this book does not allow for an exhaustive list of conditions and problems to be discussed. However, it covers some of the more common disorders that affect the modern patient.

A

Acne

Acne is a skin condition that results in redness, inflammation and cysts, often painful and infected with pus. Invariably there is an excess of the oily secretions from the skin glands (known as the sebaceous glands). They produce the necessary oils (sebum) that is vital to skin protection through keeping it waterproof and maintaining its suppleness. There are 2 types that herbalists often see: *acne vulgaris* and *acne rosacea*. The overall indication here is one of cleansing and elimination followed by modifying immune responses and examining hormonal imbalances. The symptomatic treatment can be effective and involves the use of depurative herbs such as cleavers or poke root, together with immune herbs such as echinacea or garlic and anti-inflammatories such as calendula (marigold). It is a common misconception that eating the 'wrong' foods such as chocolates, chips, cakes or biscuits are the cause but this is not the case. Although, health *per se* is not assisted in any way by eating any of these foods, and it certainly will not help the acne in any way, it is more the case that there is an immune response to a trigger and in some cases a definite hormonal imbalance. Hormonal balancers such as chaste berry (*Vitex*) are excellent in clear cases of hormonal imbalance accompanied by the symptoms of acne. There is no one single herbal formula for acne and every case is treated individually giving due regard to contributory factors, diet, lifestyle, stress & emotional states. Important supplements may include Vitamin A, Vitamin C, zinc, evening primrose oil and B-complex.

Specific topical preparations can be made to reduce the redness & inflammation, astringe the skin area affected, restore skin integrity and cleanse the area to prevent further challenge to the immune system. Herbs commonly used in skin preparations for acne may include witch hazel, calendula (marigold), vitamin E oil, lavender oil or tea tree oil. Herbalists will also look into long-term plans to treat scarring (a significant problem for many sufferers) and general management of the condition.

Addressing other factors such as stress, psychological and emotional factors are all important key areas that are examined and treated accordingly.

Allergic rhinitis – see Hayfever

Allergies

Whenever discussing this problem, it is firstly important to define what an allergy is compared to the more common intolerance. With an increasing incidence of both conditions, many people can become confused about their symptoms which can make the identification process of the cause or trigger that much more difficult. In short, an allergy is an immune response to a range of things from certain foods, pollens, pets, synthetic chemicals to prescription drugs, the living environment and toiletries to name but a few. The herbal approach is to initially identify the causative agent (referred to as allergen) and to offer comprehensive and practical advice on eliminating it or avoiding it as far as possible. The holistic aspect of treatment will examine the immune system (after all, allergy is very much an immune response) and making a thorough review of gut function. Often, many patients who are prone to allergies have a leaky gut – this means that food substances (including some waste material) pass directly through the gut wall into the tissues and spaces within the gut cavity, rather than being absorbed into the bloodstream. This has disastrous consequences for the health, not only because of possible toxic burden but also because the immune system can get to the point where it cannot cope. Combined with poor digestive function, imbalance in the gut flora, stress and other illnesses can put a heavy strain on the body resulting in immune breakdown.

Firstly, cutting out trigger foods such as dairy and wheat for example can reduce the symptoms significantly as they are known allergens. Preparing the ground for proper gut function is very important. Bitter herbs such as gentian or wormwood will improve digestive function as well as taking some probiotics (depending on the severity of the allergy) to boost gut flora. This will ensure that any toxic burden is reduced to a minimum because the gut will be able to fend off any invasion of potential allergens ingested from food. Examining digestive patterns is also critical as this will determine possible causes in cases where the allergen has not yet been identified.

The next step is to address the immune function and boost this system which has probably become overburdened with the toxic triggers on a regular basis. Herbs such as echinacea, marigold or ginseng will all boost the immune system. After this, the traditional allergy herbs such as nettle, eyebright, elderflowers, ephedra and chamomile will all address the various symptoms of allergy such as inflammation, watery and itch eyes and sneezing etc… and supplements such as quercetin and omega 3 essential fatty acids will replenish the system with the important nutrients. Supplements of butterbur (petasites) has shown favourable results in trials. A herbalist should be able to make a comprehensive review of each case and work out an individual dietary plan with specific herbal treatments for the allergy in question.

Anaemia

Many people in the West are probably anaemic without really realising it. Anaemia is really a blood disorder characterised by insufficient oxygen supply to cells and tissues. There are various types of anaemia but common symptoms include breathlessness on exertion, headaches, dizziness, fatigue, lethargy, paleness in appearance (as if all colour has been drained from the face), muscular aches and pains. The most common types are iron-deficiency anaemia and Vitamin B_{12} deficiency anaemia (also known as pernicious anaemia). Lack of sufficient oxygen supply to cells and vital organs has many consequences beyond the problem of symptoms and all its manifestations. Firstly, the type of anaemia should be identified because some anaemias require conventional treatment particularly in the acute phase (eg. sickle cell anaemia). Herbalists are more likely to see cases of iron-deficiency and Vitamin B_{12} deficiency and treatments initially focus on the causes of insufficiency.

Iron deficiency anaemia can be caused by a diet low in iron-rich foods (such as red meats, liver, dark green leafy vegetables), heavy menstrual blood loss, hidden blood loss (eg. stomach ulcer, pregnancy, bleeding piles), chronic disease (eg. liver, kidney disease or heart disease) or malnutrition in cases such as anorexia nervosa. Treatment involves simply addressing this deficiency after examining all possible causes especially hidden blood loss. Taking iron supplements can be effective but only in the short term, to eradicate an immediate physiological crisis. Long term approaches must thoroughly address diet. Herbs that are rich in iron include nettle and gentian. They can be combined with other herbs that will improve the absorption rate in addition to directly increasing iron intake into the body. These herbs are usually given as a tea. Other dietary measures should include a reduction in tea, coffee and wheat bran as they will bind together with the iron and prevent it from being absorbed into the blood. Other herbs may also be prescribed to boost energy levels and to boost digestive function, thus improving the absorption of iron. This is particularly important in the elderly since digestion becomes increasingly impaired with age.

Vitamin B_{12} deficiency anaemia is caused by a lack of vitamin B_{12} and usually occurs in middle age. In addition to the common symptoms of anaemia, distinctive features include a yellowing of the skin, failing eyesight, numbness in the legs & feet, heart problems, unsteady on the feet and depression. Treatment after initial hospitalisation to receive injections of Vitamin B_{12}, would include herbal teas containing comfrey, milk thistle, wormwood, nettle or parsley. Digestive tonics and bitters to improve stomach acid may also be advised. Supplements of B_{12} and folic acid on a short term basis may also help.

Ankylosing Spondylitis

Ankylosing spondylitis (AS) is a chronic joint disorder of the spine characterised by persistent stiffness, pain, inflammation and loss of mobility. In a manner similar to arthritis, treatment is very much a question of management. The symptomatic approach is to address the pain and any swelling so that mobility can continue. White willow bark is excellent at tackling both since it is both an anti-inflammatory and an analgesic. Herbs can be prescribed internally and/or externally as a liniment or cream. Other good herbs can include devil's claw, chamomile, celery and guaiacum. Dietary measures should include avoiding citrus fruits and to ensure sufficient intake of essential fatty acids (preferably from foods such as fatty fish, walnuts, flaxseeds, pumpkin and sunflower seeds etc...). Supplements of vitamin A, vitamin B_6, vitamin E and zinc are advisable. Taking adequate exercise is also important as this maintains mobility and suppleness in the joints. Walking, swimming, good posture, osteopathy or chiropractic are all recommended.

Anxiety

Everyone has experienced an anxious moment or two from time to time. Usually, they are triggered by a life event or distressing experience, such as a job interview, moving house, an important meeting at work or even getting back to driving after a car accident. Another overriding cause is stress. Some people worry needlessly and are often referred to as 'natural worriers' and they suffer great bouts of anxiety as a result. For such personalities, anxiety is a daily feature in their lives and dominates their very existence. Sometimes, anxiety can be present along with depression, which may be hard to imagine given that they appear opposing in their very nature. Treating anxiety requires more than a simple herbal formula and trying to understand the personality, underlying causes for the anxiety, triggers, past events or experiences can be a real challenge. Many patients benefit from counselling or psychotherapy such as CBT (cognitive behavioural therapy), particularly if depression is also a part of the condition.

Symptoms of anxiety can range from increased heartbeat, palpitations, shortness of breath, tension headaches, insomnia, weight loss, poor digestive function, increased sweating etc.... Some prefer to call this condition nervousness. Herbs that counteract anxiety are referred to as anxiolytics but often, nervines that suppress the nervous system (relaxants) can also be prescribed because they will prevent the triggering of nerves that contribute to the anxiety. Effective anxiolytics include lemon balm, passion flower, lime flowers and St. John's Wort (also an antidepressant so will be useful in patients who suffer from both anxiety and depression). Effective relaxants include chamomile, valerian (good for patients who suffer from sleep problems as a result of their anxiety), skullcap or wild lettuce. In all cases of anxiety it is extremely important to address the causes of it first before taking the herbs as an immediate solution. Much gain is to be made from reviewing experiences, however painful and discussing patterns of behaviour and the manner of responding to events. In this respect, talking therapies such as psychotherapy has great value and is particularly helpful in conjunction with herbal treatments for this condition.

Arthritis – see under Joint disorders

Asthma

Asthma is a condition characterised by the inflammation of the airways leading to obstruction of airflow into the lungs. Breathing becomes difficult and is characterised by the typical 'wheezing' sounds that are heard in asthmatics. It is an allergic response and can be to a variety of factors such as air pollution, dust mites or pets. The first approach to treating this condition is to identify the triggers and to avoid exposure to them as far as possible. The herbal treatment is essentially two-fold using bronchodilators to open up the airways, then using expectorants, antitussives (anti-cough) and demulcents to treat the symptoms such as productive cough, sore and inflamed airways.

Effective bronchodilators that are traditionally used include ephedra and lobelia. These herbs are not available as OTC medicines so it would have to prescribed by a herbalist. To soothe irritated airways would be to use demulcents such as mullein, plantain or licorice. Effective antitussives prevent the persistent coughing that can be very uncomfortable for sufferers and they include herbs such as coltsfoot or elecampane. In all asthmatics, there is the production of excess mucus which does not have the chance to clear away from the airways due to the obstruction. So a good expectorant should have the effect of encouraging the coughing up of this mucus which, if left to stay in the airways can increase the risk of chest infections which is a common symptom in sufferers. Effective expectorants include thyme, licorice and wild cherry.

Athlete's foot

Athlete's foot is caused by a fungal infection commonly referred to as ringworm. The main symptoms are itching (which can be intense at times), scaling, red and raw skin. Conditions that favour this infection are a damp, sweaty environment, made worse in warm weather and walking barefoot in places such as swimming baths, sports clubs and school gyms. People with a low resistance to infection should boost their immune system first by taking supplements like echinacea and other immune boosters. Effective anti-fungal herbs include thuja (tree of life) and poke root. Topical applications of tea tree oil or preparations including it would be beneficial. A general antiseptic such as goldenseal would also be good but a herbalists will be able to work out the best formula once they have seen the infection. Practical measures such as regular cleansing of the feet and keeping it dry and free from damp is essential. Also, using clean and protective footwear when exposed to communal areas and public sports facilities such as swimming baths is also vital.

B

Backache

Backache is one of the highest causes of sickness from work and causes endless misery to millions of sufferers. The causes of backache are many and can range from poor posture (see Chapter 5 on Health Essentials) to sports injury, arthritis, repetitive strain and pregnancy. Many sufferers seek relief from manipulation therapies such as osteopathy and chiropractic which has great value in alleviating pain and in improving mobility. It is worth considering manipulation in conjunction with herbal muscle rubs and treatments. In its simplest terms, backache can be easily treated and managed through various herbal remedies as well as massage targeted at the affected areas.

At the outset however, it is imperative to establish whether the problem lies within the joints/spine or in the muscles as this will speed up the treatment and recovery process. A proper investigation into recurring back problems is warranted in order to establish a definitive diagnosis. Herbal treatment and management focuses on reducing inflammation (if any), alleviating pain and in improving mobility. Anti-inflammatories such as devil's claw, while willow bark and St. John's Wort (applied topically) are excellent for this problem. Devil's claw and while willow bark are also effect painkillers so they are ideal herbs of choice. Topical applications of St.John's Wort oil or arnica cream have also know to be beneficial. Other notable herbs in joint conditions are prickly ash, winter green oil and cayenne pepper oil. They are better used topically as they will target the specific area more quickly and is probably better for more immediate relief. Other measures such as the Alexander Technique, pilates or yoga (as appropriate and within ability) can also help with posture and strengthen the back in order to prevent future problems.

A consultation with a herbalist is best in order to establish the cause and to work out a suitable preparation together with practical measures and other therapies as may be appropriate.

Bladder problems

Bladder problems can include BHP (benign prostatic hyperplasia), stress incontinence and a variety of bladder infections. It is not possible to discuss all the bladder conditions that people can suffer with but some of the more common ones will be discussed shortly.

BPH affects men mainly in their middle age due to an enlargement of the prostate gland. This in turn blocks the passageway for urine to pass and the condition is characterised by an constant and urgent need to pass water but proves to be difficult and there is much hesitation before doing so. Often, very little water is passed because of the blockage caused by the enlarged gland. BPH is very much a condition that is symptomatic of age and decline so very little can be done to prevent it. It is very important to have regular check ups to monitor BPH as it can sometimes be a precursor to prostate cancer. Herbal supplements of saw palmetto have shown excellent results in clinical trials. Commercial supplements are readily available but advice should be sought on brand before purchase as quality and quantity of active ingredients vary enormously. Other herbs such as buchu and damiana can be given in combination. Antioxidants of vitamins A, C and E as well as selenium are also recommended.

Stress incontinence affects more women than men, particularly if it not age-related. It is essentially regarded as bladder weakness as the control over it is reduced. Bladder instability can arise from nervous or emotional strain, coughing, sneezing or even lifting heavy weights. The most common cause in women is associated with loss of muscle tone in the sphincter that regulates the emptying of the bladder. This can happen through injury, pregnancy, birth or gynaecological problems. Herbal urinary astringents such as bearberry or horsetail are particularly good. Stress incontinence caused by psychological factors requires a thorough examination of triggers such as stressful events, anxiety and nervousness. Appropriate nervines will be prescribed by a herbalist to modify the responses to such triggers along with effective urinary astringents to deal with the distressing and often embarrassing symptoms. Other measures include appropriate exercises to strengthen and tone the pelvic muscles, ligaments and tendons that support the bladder and the sphincter muscle that regulates it.

Bladder infections are usually as a result of untreated infections of the ureter and urethra, the tubes leading up to the bladder. Symptoms include pain on passing water, discharge and in more serious infections, blood can appear in the urine. So, any treatment of the bladder should also attempt to treat the structures below it but diagnosis is essential. Those who suffer from recurring bladder infections really do not want to take repeated doses of antibiotics and we are all getting a little concerned about antibiotic resistance. Herbal urinary antimicrobials in my experience has been shown to be much more effective than taking prescription antibiotics on a regular basis for a recurring infection. It is critical to investigate the reasons why the infection has occurred as it could be sexually transmitted and the cause of the infection should be identified. In cases of non-specific infection, a range of urinary antiseptics such as bearberry, juniper berries or buchu could be advised. Cranberry juice or extracts in tablet form has proven effects and are much favoured by conventional doctors. To soothe the irritated and inflamed linings, herbs such as horsetail, couchgrass or marshmallow could be recommended. Advice needs to be sought on personal hygiene, lifestyle and nutrition especially fluid intake as are all important aspects in preventing further attacks. Some patients benefit from immune boosters such as echinacea or ginseng together with supplements of Vitamin C and zinc.

Blood disorders (eg. hypertension/high blood pressure)

Blood disorders are many and beyond the scope of this book. Anaemia has been briefly discussed. The other most common blood disorder is high blood pressure (medically referred to as hypertension). Normally there is a certain amount of resistance to the flow of blood in our blood vessels. There is an acceptable limit which is defined as normal. However, with age, a poor lifestyle and in certain disease states, the walls of the blood vessels becomes hardened and furred increasing the resistance to blood flow. This in turn, causes the heart to work much harder as it faces increasing resistance from the vessels. If the resistance exceeds the normal limits for a particular age group and physique, then this is deemed to be high blood pressure. The long term consequences of untreated hypertension can have implications for the heart, blood vessels, the kidneys, eyesight problems and the brain (risk of stroke).

In addition to age, many other factors can cause the blood pressure to rise. Smoking, a diet rich in saturated fats, excess salt, limited exercise, fluid retention and stress can all contribute to increased blood pressure. The herbal approach to combating this problem is firstly to offer proper, sensible advice about healthy eating and lifestyle changes as this alone can significantly reduce it especially if it has been caused by these factors. In some instances, herbal diuretics are effective as fluid retention can cause an increase. Good choices are celery seed, nettle, or dandelion leaf. Herbs that directly act as hypotensives ie. act directly on the blood vessels to reduce the pressure include herbs such as lime flowers, olive leaf, mistletoe or hawthorn. Garlic is also effective and has a host of other health benefits too. If the high blood pressure is caused by or made worse by stress and anxiety, then herbal relaxants or anxiolytics are advocated. Herbs such as lemon balm, passion flower, chamomile or valerian are all excellent herbs of choice. A herbalist would be able to choose the right combination of herbs together with recommendations for nutritional and lifestyle changes to combat the problem. Supplementation of vitamin C, B$_6$ or zinc to boost the health of the blood vessels may also be advised but seek help before self-medicating.

Some dietary recommendations:

- Limit salt
- Avoid processed foods and fast foods high in fat & salt (and empty calories)
- Eat cheese & meats sparingly
- Limit or avoid alcohol altogether
- Eat plenty of natural and whole foods
- Avoid tea, coffee and other stimulant drinks (eg. fizzy cola drinks)
- Switch to a more vegetable-dominant diet

Boils

A boil is a result of an infection in the skin, notably in the hair follicles and sweat glands. The affected area becomes inflamed, red and filled with pus containing dead blood cells and the bacteria. Boils are very often caused by poor personal hygiene and poor skin regimes so appropriate changes need to be made on this aspect. In some instances, it may be as a result of a diabetic state as the high sugar levels in the blood is fertile ground for all kinds of infections, particularly bacterial ones as seen in boils. It is important to rule out diabetes before starting treatment. Effective antimicrobials are echinacea, wild indigo and goldenseal. All are good at bringing the boil to the surface and counteracting the pus and infective matter by limiting the spread of infection. If the boils are recurring, then it is a matter of examining why the immune system is under constant challenge. Toxic burden on the system provokes an immune response so herbal treatments usually include depuratives to clear out the blood and tissues of the numerous toxins that challenge the immune system. Herbs such as blue flag or poke root should be beneficial in this regard as is a good lymphatic herb such as marigold (calendula). Topical preparations can include herbs such as tea tree oil or tincture of echinacea. Supplements of vitamins A, C, E and zinc are all recommended for improving and preventing infection in addition to assisting the healing process, particularly of wounds and skin eruptions.

Breast cysts (Fibrocystic breast disease)

The very nature of breast tissue means that it is prone to cysts simply because the tissue is glandular (ie. made up of mammary glands) and is under constant change on a cyclical basis. Glands are designed to secrete substances, in this case, to secrete milk. Cysts occur when there is disruption to the glandular process, invariably due to hormonal disruption and in most cases, they are harmless (ie. benign lumps). It is very important however, to keep a close check on this to make sure that it is not the forerunner to breast cancer, particularly if there is a possible risk (ie. person is a smoker or there is breast cancer in the family). In most cases also, the cysts are self-contained so their removal by surgery yields good results. On a confirmed diagnosis of benign cysts, hormonal balancers such as chaste berry (*Vitex*) or black cohosh have some value. Herbs such as poke root can also be useful as are supplements of evening primrose oil (doses of 3000mg per day) and vitamin B_6.

Bronchitis

This is a potentially serious chest infection affecting the main airways of the lungs – the bronchi. They become inflamed and congested leading to difficulty in breathing but also a risk of infection due to the build up of mucus and trapped dirt which does not clear from the airways because of the damage to their linings. Repeated attacks require a fundamental review of the causes and factors that contribute to the condition. This can range from smoking, air pollution, irritants, damp and cold living conditions. The elderly are particularly vulnerable as are those with reduced immunity who live in a heavily polluted environment as the risk of infection is greater.

Herbal approaches to treating acute episodes would be to address the symptoms and to increase immunity in order to prevent recurrence. Expectorants such as thyme, licorice or elecampane would clear the lungs and airways of the mucus (phlegm and sputum) that cause the congestion. Bronchodilators such as lobelia or ephedra would also be helpful but this can only be prescribed by a qualified, registered herbalist. This should improve breathing. Improving bloodflow with circulatory stimulants such as ginkgo or ginger to the lung surface ensures good healing but also the oxygen delivery to the cells. Herbs such as mullein or plantain will soothe the irritated linings and restore normal function so long as the cause is removed. This may involve radical steps in changing the immediate environment such as moving away from a congested and polluted environment or moving home (if possible), particularly if it is damp and cold. Important lifestyle changes such as giving up smoking is also necessary as the constant aggravation to the lining that is provoked by cigarette smoke is very much a risk factor in bronchitis. Improving resistance to infection is also vital so immune boosters such as echinacea or ginseng is advised although they will have limited effect if the cause of the damage to the airways continues to be present. This is particularly true for smokers.

Bruising

Bruising can happen for a number of reasons. It is due to injury to the tiny blood vessels near the surface of the skin (called capillaries). This can happen when there is a knock or a fall. Sometimes, the skin is left unbroken but the damage happens underneath the skin surface and the walls of the capillaries are broken and blood spills out into the nearby spaces giving the characteristic red/blue/purple appearance that is associated with a bruise. In other cases, particularly the elderly, bruising happens because the walls of their capillaries are fragile and therefore prone to damage much more easily. Healing can also take a long time and this is often true in the elderly. The herbal approach to tackling this problem is to first examine whether the skin is broken as this will affect the choice of herbs. Arnica is the classic herb of choice for bruising but it can only be applied to unbroken skin. OTC rubs, lotions and creams for bruising often contain arnica in combination with other herbs such as comfrey, chickweed, chamomile or calendula which offer some anti-inflammatory action to reduce any swelling but some healing action too. To promote the strength of the capillary walls, herbs such as bilberry are extremely good as are most bioflavonoids (provide powerful antioxidant properties) to protect and strengthen the blood vessels. Bilberry can be taken in convenient tablet form as a supplement. Horsetail is also useful as it is generally given internally for improving connective tissue strength and often prescribed for sprains, fractures and poor healing wounds. It can also benefit bruising if it is a part of the injury.

Diet is an essential part of the treatment so this is examined carefully. Supplements of Vitamin K, E ad A are advised as well foods rich in antioxidants or alternatively a good brand of bioflavonoids to boost the health of the blood vessels.

Bursitis

Quite literally, this is inflammation of the bursa, a sac-like structure made of soft, elastic tissue and containing some fluid found between the bone and the tendon. It acts like a cushion to prevent the hard surfaces from knocking against each other and to provide smooth, painless movement. It is found in joints like the elbow and shoulder. Inflammation of the bursa often occurs due to repetitive movements, wear and tear and/or overuse. It is a common sports injury.

The herbal approach to treatment is firstly to advise rest as this will prevent continuous use of the joint. As this is an inflammation, pain is often a symptom. Topical rubs containing St. John's Wort oil, comfrey, wintergreen, cayenne pepper or arnica are very useful. Other herbs given generally for rheumatic (joint) complaints such as celery, devil's claw (as supplements), white willow bark or nettle could also be used.

Supplements of Vitamins A, C and E (a good antioxidant combo) as well a turmeric tablets and zinc are also advised.

C

Candidiasis (thrush)

Thrush is a common problem and affects more women than men. The bacteria that exist in delicate balance in our system (gut flora) help protect us from illness by fighting off any invasion from foreign bacteria or other harmful pathogens. This fine balance can be easily disrupted by stress, infection illness, medication especially antibiotics, poor diet and lifestyle. Opportunistic infections take hold when the body's natural balance is upset (for whatever reason) and usually this is caused by the yeast-like fungal infection *Candida albicans*, commonly known as thrush. It usually affects the genitals and surrounding structure (vaginal thrush in women) but can also affect the gut from the mouth (oral thrush) to the lower bowel.

Symptoms of thrush can include one of more of the following: itching, burning, soreness, swelling of the vagina and vulva (outer area of the vagina), and a white, thick, yeasty-smelling discharge. Symptoms can vary from mild to severe and diagnosis is usually made on the basis of these symptoms. The herbal approach is to examine levels of immunity and to boost the numbers of the normal gut flora. Immune boosters such as goldenseal and garlic are particularly effective in thrush. Topical application of a good anti-fungals such as calendula or tea tree oil (as pessary, cream or gel) counteract the fungal infection and soothe the affected areas. Aloe vera gel is particularly soothing to sore and inflamed linings. A good probiotic combination of *Lactobacilli* and *Bifidobacteria* should boost the levels of normal gut flora and so restore the delicate balance within the system. Dietary measures include cutting out or eliminating as far as possible any foods containing yeast and increase intake of yoghurts containing *lactobacillus*. In severe cases, a restricted diet eliminating sugar and yeast-based products are advised for at least 3 months. Personal hygiene measures include avoiding the use of soaps, detergents, cleansers and perfumes that strip the area of essential oils and bacteria in that area is advised as they may do more harm than good.

Carpel tunnel syndrome (RSI)

This is a condition characterised by pain and swelling. It is often categorised under RSI or repetitive strain injury because one of the causes may be due to over-activity of the part of the hand relating to the relevant structures. In essence, one of the many nerves that supply the hand goes through a sheath-like structure shaped like a tunnel and is located at the wrist. Through a variety of causes (overuse being one of them), the sheath gets inflamed and swollen, leading to pain, numbness, tingling and loss of mobility due to muscle weakness. Other causes can include injury, joint disorders in the hand, overuse of the computer keyboard, vibrating mechanical power tools, musical instruments or video games and in some cases, tumours. In other cases, the cause is simply due to anatomical differences, namely that the wrist is small and therefore the aperture through which the nerves can be passed via the carpal tunnel is narrowed, increasing the pressure on the nerves. Underlying causes such as diabetes, hypothyroidism or arthritis have to be ruled out prior to treatment. Conventional treatments rely on drugs (painkillers and anti-inflammatories), specific exercises to restore the mobility and strength of the muscles affected and surgery. After a definitive diagnosis, herbal treatments are carried out within the holistic context that explores the cause in some detail. Addressing causes such as overuse, overactivity or injury quite simply involves either eliminating it or limiting it as far as possible. Supplements of Vitamin B$_6$, Vitamin C, bromelain, turmeric are all useful as are topical herbal creams containing St. John's Wort oil, chamomile or cramp bark. Internal mixtures containing centella or horsetail are also good as they will encourage connective tissue repair and healing. Other therapies such as acupuncture, chiropractic or yoga have also proved to be beneficial.

Catarrh

Catarrh is the unpleasant accumulation of excess mucus from the inflammation of the mucous membranes in the nose and throat. Constant challenges from environmental pollution, an allergic response, smoking or infection results in this excessive production that becomes difficult to clear away and can obstruct the airways and make breathing difficult. Common causes range from food (intolerance or allergy), dust and dietary deficiency. Herbal treatments are tailor made for each patient so identifying the cause or factors that make it worse is the first line treatment protocol. If it is infective, then good immune boosters and antimicrobials such as wild indigo, goldenseal or garlic are advised. Gargles and inhalations containing myrrh, tea tree, mint or eucalyptus are all helpful in improving breathing in cases of nasal congestion. Anti-catarrhal herbs for the chest include solidago, plantain, ephedra and mullein.

Catarrh can also affect other organs such as the gut, bladder or lungs so getting to the root cause of excessive mucus production and congestion is a priority before commencing treatment and this become more important if the problem is recurring or chronic.

Chilblains

Chilblains are due to an abnormal reaction to the cold. The extremities such as the fingers and toes are commonly affected resulting in raised, red, itchy, swollen patches on the exposed areas of the skin. Chilblains usually go away within a week or so but it is essential to keep warm and to wrap up well when going out into the cold. It is not clear why some people are more prone to chilblains than others but it is highly likely that poor circulation plays a part. Good circulation relies on good nutrition and regular exercise. Herbal circulatory stimulants such as cayenne pepper, ginger, garlic or ginkgo have an important role in boosting blood flow near the skin surface, particularly at the extremities. Equally, herbs that support blood flow from the heart are also useful as they will improve overall circulation. In this respect, herbs such as hawthorn, bilberry or prickly ash are particularly effective. Addressing nutritional deficiencies is a must. Of particular importance is calcium, the B vitamins and vitamin E. A good bioflavonoid supplement containing an antioxidant combination of vitamins A, C and E is recommended to boost the health of the blood vessels.

Chronic Fatigue Syndrome (CFS)

CFS is technically known as myalgic encephalomyelitis or ME for short. In its literal sense, ME is the swelling of the brain and spinal cord. Symptoms include a marked and prolonged fatigue lasting up to 6 months or more with no identifiable cause and typically with a flu-like illness. There is general muscle weakness and pain with low grade fever, sore throat, painful swellings of the glands, particularly in the neck and armpits. The fatigue is worse after moderate or strenuous exercise lasting as long as a day or more. Other symptoms can include joint pain, confusion, irritability, non-refreshing sleep, poor concentration, memory loss and eyesight problems. The cause of CFS is not yet known although it has been associated with nutritional deficiencies, viral infection and fungal infection. The herbal approach to treatment or management of CFS is a complex undertaking that involves a detailed case history examining things from diet, lifestyle and influences of stress to making a thorough assessment of the psychological and mental well-being. The main symptoms of pain and fatigue can be addressed using analgesics such as cramp bark or valerian for the pain and stimulants such as rosemary or oats are particularly effective. Siberian ginseng is recommended for coping with stress as this can contribute to the symptoms. Graded aerobic exercise programmes have shown some promise in muscle fatigue and pain as does Cognitive Behavioural Therapy (CBT) and counselling.

Other approaches can include acupuncture which may alleviate muscle pain. Practical measures such as stress reduction techniques, meditation, biofeedback or joining a self-help group are all helpful. Gentle exercises such as yoga, swimming, Tai Chi or slow walking is advocated following a period of initial rest. Dietary changes should include wholefoods, raw foods if possible, organic and animal-free (for general detoxification and to reduce the toxic burden on the system), foods to improve the immune system and those that would rebalance the acid-base equilibrium in the blood. Elimination of refined carbohydrates, caffeine and alcohol is recommended in addition to increased consumption of organically grown fruits and vegetables. Additionally, food allergies and intolerances such as *Candida albicans* feature heavily and special diets are devised for those patients. A consultation with a medical herbalist is strongly advised to consider all aspects in each case.

Circulation problems

Circulation problems can be many, ranging from poor circulation, bruising, varicose veins and muscle cramps to dizziness or digestive symptoms. In simple terms the strength and resilience of the blood vessels in addition to a healthy, robust heart is the key to good circulation. It is equally important to examine the causes of circulatory problems and this can be varied from diet to lifestyle, housing conditions and infection to genetic predisposition. A healthy heart is utterly dependent on diet and exercise. Poor lifestyle habits such as excessive alcohol intake and smoking are also limiting factors to a healthy heart. Circulation of blood from the heart is dependent on the strength of the heart muscles. Herbs that are considered heart tonics boost this function and encourage a better force of contraction of the heart muscles. In cases of a weakened heart, herbs of choice include hawthorn or motherwort. Other notable herbs include the lesser perwinkle and ginkgo, both of which are also excellent for improving blood flow to the brain and surrounding organs. Grapeseed or grape vine is good for improving capillary resistance so it is good for constitutions that are prone to bruising. If there is a tendency to feeling the cold due to poor circulation to the extremities, then herbs such as ginger, cinnamon and ginkgo are all excellent as they will improve blood flow to these areas and the smaller blood vessels near the surface of the skin.

Cold sores

Cold sores are caused by a combination of a susceptible immune system, exposure to sunlight as a trigger and type 1 of the *herpes simplex* virus. It is uncertain why some people are more prone to it than others but it is believed that approximately 80 per cent of the adult population have antibodies against this type of virus in their blood with about a quarter of them experiencing recurrent attacks of cold sores throughout their lives. The primary infection can progress in different ways. Some people only have very mild symptoms or none at all. The first outbreak starts one to three weeks after the virus has been contracted. It subsides spontaneously within a few weeks. A flare up of the infection can result in intense, painful sores that produce crusting slam blisters. This is around the line of the mouth affecting the mucous membranes of the lips. Sometimes, it can also affect the mucous membranes of the nose.

There are a number of commercial OTC treatments that can soothe and heal but does not effectively tackle the root cause of this infection. Preventing recurrent attacks is the desired outcome for all patients and usually, they have a very good idea of the early warning signs of an impending attack. Long-term measures should involve a thorough examination of diet and general immunity. Getting plenty of sleep and adequate exercise is also essential.

Herbal treatments usually include immune boosters such as echinacea or ginseng. Good anti-viral herbs such as lemon balm or St. John's Wort are versatile since they can be used both internally (in tincture form) or topically in creams (essential oil of lemon balm, fixed oil of St. John's Wort). Equally, tea tree oil is excellent as it is a potent anti-viral herb and is one the few essential oils that can be used neat onto the skin. Herbalists will usually add tea tree oil to the preparation as a combination treatment. Supplements of Vitamin C and zinc in addition to an amino acid called lysine is also recommended as is observing strict personal hygiene in order to minimise complications with bacterial infections or its spread to other parts of the body. Limiting skin exposure to strong sunlight is also recommended.

Cold/flu

Almost everyone has experienced a cold. It is caused by the common cold virus. And because there are so many varieties of the cold virus (symptoms they produce are very similar as they follow the typical immune response), it is almost impossible to find a cure for it. Fewer people however have experienced the flu (influenza) and is often classed together with the common cold even though the cause of this is known. The flu vaccine is now routinely prescribed and administered to the elderly, other vulnerable groups (eg. child flu vaccine) and health care practitioners who come into direct contact with patients. Whether this is an effective measure remains debatable.

The most effective intervention for patients is in preventing frequent or recurring bouts of the common cold. In this situation, it is almost certainly the case that the immune system is weakened and is compromised to a very great extent. There are other factors at play here such as diet, stress and adrenal exhaustion, emotional health, exposure to infection and deficiency states. The herbal approach aims to tackle the holistic context in which recurring colds occur. This involves a thorough examination of all the factors mentioned above and tailor make a remedy as a long-term measure in boosting immunity, making the system more robust to infection and perhaps addressing underlying causes such as psychological well-being, the emotional health and lifestyle factors.

Immune boosting herbs such as ginseng and wild indigo are excellent. Echinacea is best taken as a prophylactic and people often take it when it is too late being disappointed at the lack of impact. A herbalist will be able to advise on reputable brands or better still tailor make a formula for improving non-specific immunity and making the system more robust at combating infection. Symptomatic treatment such as a fever, runny nose, inflammation etc…can all be addressed through general herb action such as elderflower, chamomile and mint. These are best taken as a soothing tea. Coughs are best addressed through taking syrups containing thyme, licorice or wild cherry. Supplements of Vitamin C and zinc have also been shown to be useful in people with immune deficiency.

Colic, flatulence & bloating

Colic is characterised by spasms of the muscles found in the walls, invariably of a hollow organ such as the stomach. It can also occur in the kidneys, caused by obstruction (often a stone) resulting in excruciating pain and considerable discomfort. Colic of the gut is equally uncomfortable and sometimes it is accompanied by flatulence (excessive gas and trapped air) and bloating (distension of the abdomen). All three symptoms are indicative of poor digestive function or a bad diet. Stress, anxiety and emotional distress can also wreak havoc on gut function as can any disruption to the gut flora (healthy bacteria that normally reside in delicate balance) resulting in abnormal numbers of unhealthy bacteria, spasms of the gut wall and the production of excessive gas. Age, infection and lifestyle can also be highly significant as can the symptoms of stomach ulcers and IBS, which needs to be ruled out before commencing treatment.

The herbal approach to dealing with these set of symptoms is to thoroughly examine all factors especially diet and lifestyle. Herbs to soothe the gut wall (demulcents) in addition to herbs that counteract the spasms (antispasmodics) are usually recommended. These would include chamomile, sweet flag or angelica. For the bloating, herbs such as fennel, aniseed or ginger, taken in combination as a tea provides excellent relief. In order to redress the bacterial imbalance, herbs such as goldenseal or turmeric are good as they will combat any infection. This should be taken in combination with supplements of a good probiotic. Additionally, soothing herbs of licorice or slippery elm to line the gut in cases of any inflammation may provide temporary relief. However, important dietary and/or lifestyle modifications may be necessary. Emotional or psychological aspects (stress, anxiety etc…) all need attention. Good anxiolytics such as lemon balm, passion flower or chamomile may be useful but some may benefit from talking therapies (eg. psychotherapy or CBT) if the underlying cause is more deep rooted that only such intervention will truly address the symptoms.

Constipation

This can be defined as the unduly infrequent and difficult emptying of the bowels. The person has to strain which leads to pain and sometimes rupture of the small blood vessels in the anal wall. This is referred to as piles (haemorrhoids) which is a common complication of constipation. It is almost unheard of in people with a high fibre diet, a healthy, well-balanced diet and in vegetarians who eat a high proportion of insoluble fibre.

The herbal approach would be to examine the diet thoroughly but constipation can also be a symptom of other underlying problems such as an underactive thyroid, medication (especially iron supplements prescribed for anaemia), pregnancy, lack of fluids, IBS, abuse of laxatives, problems with the gut itself (eg. obstruction) or other serious disorders. Identifying the cause is critical as the treatment may involve treating this as a primary cause of the condition.

For dietary causes and as a temporary measure in treating the symptoms, herbal laxatives are prescribed in conjunction with other useful herbs. They vary in potency and are chosen carefully depending on the severity of the problem being treated. However, long-term prescription of herbal laxatives is not usually common practice since prescription of any herbal medicines will be accompanied by comprehensive dietary advice, modifications and recommendations. Notable herbal laxatives such as senna, rhubarb and buckthorn bark are very useful in enhancing the elimination process in the gut. Additionally, bulking agents such as flaxseeds (eg. sprinkled over cereals or in salads) or psyllium husks (eg. mixed with fruit juices or smoothies) are very beneficial and better for long-term use when incorporated into the daily diet.

Crohn's disease

Crohn's disease comes under the category of the Inflammatory Bowel Diseases, the other one being Ulcerative Colitis (UC). Crohn's is very similar to UC and to distinguish the two has often proved difficult for clinicians because of the large crossover of symptoms in the two conditions. Crohn's disease is a chronic inflammation of the bowel, affecting any part of it from the mouth to the anus, though it is usually the latter part of it (large intestine) that is frequently affected. It is sometimes characterised by persistent ulcerations which over time repair and heal. Persistent ulcerations continue to damage the gut lining and a cycle of inflammation and healing leads to scar formation which can narrow the gut aperture. This leads to obstruction in parts of the gut and the dietary consequences can be severe, sometimes requiring surgery to remove part of the affected gut. It is a very distressing condition for patients, particularly during acute episodes that are characterised by pain, gut obstruction, bleeding and possible malnutrition.

The herbal approach is really one of management and often interspersed with care within mainstream medicine during acute episodes. Herbal anti-inflammatories have a lot to offer in soothing irritated and inflamed linings of the gut mucosa. Chamomile and marshmallow as a tea is particularly useful in this regard. Fenugreek seeds are usually given, sometimes soaked in water overnight. Fenugreek tea is prepared by soaking 500 mg of the seed in about 5 ounces of cold water for at least 3 hours. The seeds are then strained out of the liquid before drinking the tea, which can be heated or ingested cold. Fenugreek contains a substantial amount of mucilaginous fibre which does not dissolve but instead swells when mixed with fluids. Since the body cannot digest the mucilage from fenugreek it is believed to be an effective laxative. It can also be taken in tincture form (3-4ml three times a day). Other useful herbs are tormentil, goldenseal, licorice and meadowsweet which can be given in tincture form as a mixture. They will help reduce the inflammation and encourage healing of the mucous membranes in the gut thereby causing a soothing effect.

For cracks or ulcers at the corners of the mouth (a classic hallmark of Crohn's), topical creams containing comfrey, chamomile and marigold base creams combined with fixed oils of centella and hemp seed is particularly effective in restoring skin integrity and reducing inflammation. A longer term management approach would have to consider the immune system as this could be defective in this condition. Immune modulators such as echinacea are excellent choices but a consultation with a herbalist is necessary to formulate an individual prescription in specific cases.

Cystitis

Cystitis is an inflammation of the urinary tract system caused by a bacterial infection. It can affect any part of the system from the passage leading from the bladder to the outside of the body (urethra) or the tubes leading from the kidneys to the bladder (ureter). The latter is potentially more serious as this may involve further infection that could affect kidney function. Immediate treatment should be sought. It affects more women than men because the urethras in women are much shorter than in men and the risk of infection from the external environment is therefore much higher in women. Infection can arise due to poor personal hygiene, sexual intercourse or general immune deficiency. It is also possible in post menopausal women due to the lack of moisture in the vagina and surrounding mucous membranes, leading to dry skin that can tear, leaving it exposed to infection.

The herbal approach is to address all outside factors in addition to combating the infection. Herbal antimicrobials that are particularly suited to urinary tract infections (UTI) include cranberry (good as a powder, dissolved in water or as supplements), bearberry or goldenrod. Urinary demulcents provide relief by soothing the irritated linings; herbs that are useful here would be cornsilk or couchgrass. An alkaline diet is also advised. General tonic herbs for the urinary system includes nettle which is best drunk as a tea. Another useful antimicrobial is juniper berries which can be conveniently taken as a supplement. A herbalist would prepare the best formula and preparation type which will take into account lifestyle and a susceptibility to this type of infection. They may prescribe a general all-round immune booster as well as provide advice on dietary and/or lifestyle changes that may be impacting on the frequency of the episodes. Personal hygiene and safe sexual practices are also discussed.

D

Dandruff

Dandruff is described as the excessive flaking of dead skin cells from the scalp. It is often quite visible and people experiencing this problem are often embarrassed by it. It is normal for skin cells to shed dead cells which slough off and this flaking of dead skin cells is not usually visible in most people because the numbers are relatively small. However, in others there is a rapid turnover of skin cells in the scalp for one reason or another, maturing and shedding within 2-7 days.

There have been a number of suggestions as to the cause of dandruff from fungal infections, sugar and allergic reactions to hair products and by-products of other types of micro-organisms that reside in the hair/scalp. The most compelling evidence is in a type of fungal infection but it is dependent on other factors such as the oily secretion in the skin and individual susceptibility.

There is much to be gained from conventional anti-dandruff treatment which contains specific anti-fungal agents. Preventing further recurrence can be addressed through other means. Due to the excessive dryness of this condition, the herbal approach would be to nourish the hair by replenishing it with the essential oils that are necessary for good skin health (and that includes the scalp). Dandruff is essentially an immune response so modulating this requires herbs such as echinacea. An important part of this approach is through nutrition which aims to ensure adequate intakes of essential fatty acids (omega 3, 6 and 9) found in food sources such as fish oils (particularly fatty fish such as salmon, mackerel, trout, herring and tuna), flaxseed oil and hemp seed oil. Nuts such as walnuts, sunflower seeds and pumpkin seeds also contain the oils. Equally topical treatments of avocado oil can be massaged into the scalp and left to soak in before shampooing. This should be done on a on a regular basis for a few weeks to some months.

Herbal hair rinses containing dried sage, rosemary or thyme steeped in warm apple cider vinegar base has been shown to offer some relief to sufferers mainly because these herbs have potent anti-fungal properties. The vinegar helps restore the hair's correct pH. The hair rinse is applied after shampooing. Dandruff should be clearly distinguished from psoriasis and from seborrhoeic dermatitis. A consultation with a herbalist is highly recommended.

Debility – see under 'Weakeness and Debility'

Dehydration
Most of us have a dehydrated system without realising it. Modern living alone is enough to deplete our systems of adequate water. However, many of us are probably unaware of how much water we should drink every day in order for our cells to be fully functional. The dangerous consequences of not drinking enough water is that we lose concentration, our skin become dry and prone to other problems as a result (including infection), lethargy, fatigue, dizziness, nausea and possibly vomiting in serious cases, nerve problems, mental and psychological disturbances to name but a few. The nutritional consequences are endless but simply put, inadequate intake of water can affect digestion and absorption of nutrients. Long-term consequences lead to more the more serious effects of nutritional deficiencies through poor breakdown of food and poor absorption of nutrients.

The treatment is simple – ensure adequate intakes of water every day (approx. 2 litres per day, and possibly more during high activity). In the short term, possible nutritional deficiencies should be addressed through taking a good all round multivitamin and mineral supplement switching to fresh food sources after a few weeks. Adding a teaspoon of each salt and sugar to a glass of water in severe cases of dehydration will restore some of the lost electrolytes and ensure the correct levels of chemicals in the system as well as the correct pH balance.

Depression
Almost everyone has suffered from some form of depression at one time or another in their lives. The current UK statistic of 1 in 4 being affected by this condition is set to soon increase to 1 in 3. There are different types and various reasons for their cause. Some have clinical depression which can be a constitutional

manifestation and this requires professional help, mostly through conventional means. In other serious cases, people can suffer from schizophrenia, sometime being accompanied by violent outbursts through to self-harm and suicide.

The majority of us have suffered from mild to moderate depression at some time or another. A common cause can be a lack of sunlight giving rise to SAD (seasonally affected disorder). As the term implies, this type of depression is more common during the winter months than at any other time in the year. Sometimes, depression can be reactional, that is, it is triggered by a life event such as divorce, bereavement, post-natal or a stressful incident. A large proportion of depression in the western world is merely due to lifestyle and the stresses of modern living.

Treating depression is a complex undertaking and proper help is strongly recommended either from the doctor or from talking therapies such as counselling. There are a number of herbal antidepressants which are effective for mild to moderate depression. Establishing the cause of it and exploring the context of the illness is a vital consideration. Many have gained the benefits of St. John's Wort but other herbs such as damiana, lemon balm, passion flower and some nerviness are equally useful, particularly in addressing any nervous tension or anxiety. Sleep is profoundly affected too so herbal sedatives such as chamomile or valerian will be considered.

Addressing nutritional needs is a must as often patients neglect this first simply because they lack the motivation to cook, to shop or to eat proper, wholesome foods. Assessing any deficiency states is a priority and short term measures through supplementation can serve a useful purpose. However, proper nutritional advice as a long term measure is usually given. Foods such as porridge oats are especially nourishing to the nervous system. Limiting caffeine, refined sugars and processed foods is also advised. Increasing intake of spinach, whole grains, legumes such alfalfa, clover, the pulses, lentils, beans, lupins, peas and peanuts are particularly advised as they will be high in vitamin B which is essential for a healthy nervous system. Ensuring adequate intakes of iron (red meats, liver, eggs, spinach, chick peas, dried figs or apricots are good sources) and calcium (milk and other dairy products, spinach, fish, dark green vegetables such as broccoli and kale are good sources). Essential fatty acids with high omega 3 fatty acid (fish oils, flaxseed oil, hemp seed) is a useful supplement in depression. It can also be obtained in fresh foods such as fatty fish, walnuts and baked winter squash.

Other measures such as stress management, counselling, relaxation techniques, exposure to sunlight and exercise are all advised. A consultation with a medical herbalist is strongly recommended.

Dermatitis

Dermatitis is described as an inflammatory reaction to any cause ranging from a chemical substance, to an innocuous agent (eg. a toiletry product), possibly an allergen, an irritant or a pollutant. It is characterised by redness, blistering of the skin, swelling, weeping, crusting and itching. It is non-specific condition and part of large number of inflammatory disorders. Specific causes can result in contact dermatitis, in which the cause can be known through the pattern of inflammation which identifies the contact with the culprit substance. Seborrhoeic dermatitis is local inflammation resembling severe dandruff. Again, there is redness, scales, crusting, yellowish patches and itching. It affects mainly the scalp, eyebrows, beard area and groins. In very young children, this is referred to as cradle cap.

Herbal treatments for general dermatitis includes anti-inflammatories such as chamomile, anti-pruritic (anti-itch) agents such as chickweed cream or applying aloe vera gel to soothe and calm the skin. The herbalists' approach is one of elimination of the toxins that are triggering the body's immune system. The approach is therefore one of using depuratives such as blue flag or burdock, combined with immune modulators such as echinacea. Other useful herbs used are poke root, chamomile, sarsparilla and centella. Some of these herbs also help restore skin integrity. Due to the allergic nature of the response, nettles are also useful, particularly combined as a tea with chamomile, dandelion and alfalfa. A good circulatory stimulant such as ginkgo is also given to improve blood flow to the area and to help with skin healing.

Supplements such as vitamin C and zinc are useful as is a good vitamin B complex. In those where there is a stomach acid deficiency, a supplement of betaine hydrochloride is suggested. Most dry skin conditions will also benefit from a good supplement of the essential fatty acids such as fish oils or flaxseed oil for their omega 3 content.

Diabetes

There are different forms of diabetes but the most common one brought on through lifestyle and poor diet is the non-insulin dependent diabetes mellitus (NIDDM or type 2 diabetes). It usually manifests mid to late life (also termed late onset diabetes for this reason) but it is getting more common in the younger population, particularly in children. The increasing incidence of childhood obesity is partly to blame for this. NIDDM is essentially the inability of the body to regulate blood sugar levels owing to the insufficiency of insulin secretion or the cells' unresponsiveness to it. The latter is a condition brought on by long-term exposure to persistently raised sugar levels resulting in persistently raised insulin levels so much so that the cells eventually fail to respond to the hormone. This metabolic disorder is called Syndrome X (the pre-diabetic state also known as insulin resistance) and is the precursor to other more serious life-threatening conditions such as heart disease, high blood pressure and stroke, not to mention the complications through diabetes.

NIDDM can be managed effectively through herbal treatments and through diet and lifestyle. As the term implies, it is not dependent on injections of insulin and the key role of herbs is to improve blood sugar control and reduce the need for insulin or hypoglycaemic drugs.

Herbs of choice such as fenugreek and goat's rue are both effective hypoglycaemics directly combating the high sugar levels where pancreatic activity is still present but is significantly reduced. Fenugreek seeds have to be soaked first before being taken as a liquid preparation. Similarly bitter melon or bitter gourd is a popular vegetable in the Asian subcontinent, parts of Africa and South America but it is the extracted juice that is administered as a drink. Studies show that it controls the production of insulin, thus promoting blood sugar control. Good commercial preparations can now be bought in good health food stores. The juice is potently bitter but it is this very bitterness that combats the cravings for sweet foods. Sugar cravings can be equally addressed through taking gymnema, a herb that temporarily anaesthetises the taste buds corresponding to sweet foods. Consequently, foods that are high in sugar cannot be tasted and thus the addictive consumption of foods with a high sugar content is reduced. For this reason, gymnema must be administered in liquid form on the tongue since tablet or capsule form exert no therapeutic effect. Gymnema is particularly effective in mild cases of diabetes.

The main use of herbs in type 2 diabetes is to prevent the long term complications. In this respect the following herbs are useful:

- **Diabetic retinopathy** (eye symptoms) - extracts of bilberry, gingko or grapeseed. All contain significant levels of flavonoids (anthocyanidins and proanthocyanidins). Flavonoids are noted for their beneficial effects on capillaries

- **Infections** – echinacea or astragalus to boost non-specific immunity as well as to combat infection directly

- **Risk of CHD** (coronary heart disease) –turmeric, hawthorn or lime flowers are all indicated where there is accompanying high blood pressure

- **Boost pancreatic health** – *Taraxacum officinale* (dandelion), *Siliybum marianum* (milk thistle) are also good liver herbs that have a positive effect on the pancreas

- **Dietary interventions** ↑ complex carbohydrates
  ↑ fibre
  ↓ trans fatty acids, saturated fats & salt

- **Increase intake of foods that ↑ insulin production:**
  Banana
  Barley,
  Cabbage
  Lettuce
  Oats
  Olive
  Papaya
  Turnip
  Sweet potato

Diabetes has a complex clinical presentation resulting from an altered glucose metabolism. It can be destructive and debilitating in the long-term, particularly if it goes undiagnosed and untreated for many years. Diet, environment and lifestyle all contribute to this condition and equal emphasis should be placed on reducing the incidence of childhood obesity that predisposes the system to NIDDM at a very young age. Early diagnosis is essential in preventing the long-term complications of NIDDM, particularly heart disease, stroke, kidney disease and associated disorders involving the eyes and the nervous system. A consultation with a medical herbalist is highly recommended before self-medicating.

Diarrhoea

Diarrhoea is characterised by increased bowel movement caused by an infection, an intense emotional or psychological response, medication or a food intolerance. Due to the rapid nature of transit, the bowel does not have enough time to absorb water so the stools end up being watery and loose. People suffering from diarrhoea need to be very careful not to get dehydrated as a result, especially children. To replace important electrolytes and sugar, it is best to add a teaspoon each of salt and sugar to each glass of water.

Infective causes need to be investigated properly and an examination of food handling, food preparation and food hygiene may need to be reviewed. The best course of action for diarrhoea in the short term is to drink plenty of water to prevent dehydration which if left unattended can lead to more serious problems. Switching to a bland diet will also help although in cases of food poisoning, it is best not to eat much until the diarrhoea has stopped. Restoring the numbers of 'friendly' bacteria is important after an acute episode because this will prevent susceptibility and further attack by promoting healthy numbers of good bacteria to combat any pathogenic ones. A good combination probiotic that includes acidophilus (*Lactobacillus* species) and bifidus (*Bifidobacterium* species) are highly recommended.

The herbal approach is to provide some immediate relief through astringents. A cup of black tea (brewed for a good 5 minutes) can help. Herb teas made from agrimony, walnut leaves, peppermint leaves, tormentil and chamomile should be drunk for the first few days until the gut has calmed down. Ginger capsules can address any lingering infection as well as soothe the gut and peppermint oil (2 drops morning and evening) can be taken as a preventative measure.

Restoring the lining of the gut after a bout of diarrhoea is also important. In this respect slippery elm powder or aloe vera (not the juice as this has laxative properties) can prove useful. Dietary measures should address the causes especially if there is a food intolerance. Diarrhoea of psychological origin requires special help through talking therapies such as counselling or cognitive behavioural therapy (CBT). Persistent or recurring diarrhoea should always be properly examined. It is important to distinguish the diarrhoea from other problems such as the inflammatory bowel diseases (Crohn's disease and ulcerative colitis) as well as irritable bowel syndrome (IBS). In the older patient, particularly the elderly, it is best to get a proper check from the GP to rule out bowel cancer or other serious problems.

Duodenal ulcers

A duodenal ulcer is an inflammation of the gut lining (at the region of the duodenum) caused by acid infiltration through a normally mucus-protected lining. In some, there is insufficient mucus being produced so the normal levels of protection against the acid is no longer present and this results in ulceration of the gut lining, specifically at the point of the duodenum, hence the term duodenal ulcer. The symptoms are intermittent abdominal pain, sometimes eased by eating but often patients are woken up from their sleep as a result of this pain. Other symptoms include bloating, retching, nausea and a feeling of being extremely 'full' especially after meals. In some cases, eating may make the pain worse. In more serious cases, the complications arise from rupture of the gut wall (perforation) after prolonged bleeding leading to anaemia in the first instance. Thereafter, food and acid from the gut leak into the abdominal cavity causing severe pain and life-threatening toxicity (peritonitis). This is a medical emergency and will require immediate assistance.

The causes of duodenal ulcers are varied but in most of the cases there is an infection of *Helicobacter pylori*. This bacterium affects the lining of the duodenum, in some way that is poorly understood, enabling the acid to cause inflammation and ulceration. Other causes include anti-inflammatory medication especially the non-steroidal anti-inflammatory drugs (NSAIDs) such as aspirin, ibuprofen and diclofenec. It is thought that these medicines somehow affect the duodenal lining allowing the acid to cause inflammation and ulceration. Other factors such as smoking, stress and heavy drinking may increase the risk of duodenal ulcers but it is not predominantly the underlying cause of them.

Due to the very nature of ulcers, it is best to give herbal medicines as a tea or dissolved powders. Herbal teas made from marshmallow, meadowsweet, plantain, chamomile and slippery elm are particularly effective. Slippery elm can also be taken in convenient tablet form especially at night time to prevent acid attack, or the powdered bark can be added to the tea mixture. Making certain lifestyle changes will also help by not exacerbating the condition. A consultation with a medical herbalist is highly recommended.

Dysbiosis

This term refers to the general disruption of the balance of normal gut bacteria that reside in the system in order to fend off other invaders. These bacteria are termed 'friendly' bacteria because of this function. Any imbalance to the ratio between good and bad bacteria can lead to a variety of common symptoms such as thrush, a whole host of digestive complaints (eg. bloating, flatulence and indigestion), headaches and joint pains to name but a few. Other infections that can also take hold because the healthy bacteria are not in sufficient numbers to fight off the harmful ones.

The causes of dysbiosis vary from over use of antibiotics, other medication, chronic illness, stress, infection and poor diet. The treatment needs to start off by identifying and eliminating the cause of the imbalance. Infection can be treated with immunostimulants such as the ginsengs, echinacea or wild indigo, depending on the cause. These herbs will also boost general immunity to prevent further attack although other factors have to be addressed as well. Restoring healthy numbers of the normal bacteria found in the gut is the next step and a good probiotic supplement should address that. Ensure that the supplement contains acidophilus (*Lactobacillus* sp) and bifidus (*Bifidobacterium* sp) as these two types are very important for healthy gut function.

Avoid yeast-type foods especially white bread, white rice, fruits at the beginning especially bananas and switch to whole foods as far as possible. Cut down on refined sugars and simple carbohydrates, opt for vegetables, whole grains, pulses and complex carbohydrates. Limit stimulants such as tea, coffee and cut down on alcohol. Drink plenty of water and take regular exercise as this will boost immunity and improve circulation. Limit high protein foods especially animal flesh, increase intakes of fermented dairy products such as yoghurt and other milk products.

Herbal supplements of garlic, goldenseal or barberry are all excellent choices. Healing the gut and preparing the lining is assisted by slippery elm. It is best taken as a powder but many may find that taking tablets of it more convenient. Alternatively it can be added to a herbal tea containing herbal relaxants and anxiolytics to address any stress. Good choices would be chamomile, passion flower and lemon balm.

E

Ear disorders

Ear disorders are many and can range from earache and ear infection to hearing impairment or loss of hearing. A common problem is 'ringing in the ears', medically referred to as tinnitus. The causes of any ear disorder have to be thoroughly investigated and defined before any treatment can be considered. In this respect, a proper examination needs to be carried out either by a GP or a herbalist.

Another common ear disorder is excessive ear wax in the outer ear. This leads to hearing impairment or in severe cases, hearing loss. The cause of wax build up should always be considered in any symptom with hearing loss. Ear wax is essential for proper hearing as the sound waves bounce off these to create a clear reverberation before it reaches the eardrum. It also traps dirt, small insects and dust and this keeps the rest of the ear structure clear of foreign material and harmful agents.

In healthy cases, ear wax clears away naturally but in others, it stagnates and this may increase the chances of infection. OTC wax softening drops may provide immediate relief in mild cases but does not address the root cause of the accumulation. A more natural approach is to use a couple of drops of warmed (body temperature) olive oil or garlic oil into the ear two or three times a day, for a few days. After three or four days the ears can be washed out by a nurse or other health care practitioner. If there is a hole in the ear drum (a perforation), it is not advisable to put drops in your ear without having first discussed it with your doctor or a competent medical advisor.

If there is ear pain or a raised temperature, there is a possibility of an infection, particularly if there is a pus being produced which may drain out of the ear. This requires immediate treatment either conventionally or using herbal medicines (see earache below).

Any infection of the outer ear is potentially a problem and must be treated immediately before it spreads to other parts of the ear or get worse. It is often termed 'swimmer's ear' as it is swimmers who frequently get outer ear infections. Causes are either bacterial or fungal infections acquired when swimming as are dirty fingernails, excessive sweating, poor skin hygiene, eczema or diabetes. Herbal treatments include a good antimicrobial such as echinacea, garlic, astralagus or goldenseal combined with circulatory stimulants such as ginkgo or ginger. A good demulcent will soothe and calm the skin and topical preparations containing licorice or chamomile cream with centella oil will help heal the area.

Tinnitus is another common problem affecting the ears although the cause may originate in the head. The sound is usually only heard by the person affected by it and it can be a hissing, whistling, clicking or ringing sound appearing to come from one or both ears. It is usually associated with deafness although it can be caused by anything that damages the hearing mechanism of the inner ear such as loud noise, toxic drugs to the ears and diseases that cause ear nerve damage. The causes are many and varied but it can also be associated with ear wax and catarrh.

Herbal approaches will examine the underlying causes first. For catarrh, dietary modifications such as limiting dairy foods, refined foods, alcohol and caffeine etc. are advised. Drinking lots of mineral water and doing more things to relax is also recommended. There have been good results with ginkgo as with nervines for the stressed and anxious patients. In this respect, herbs such as skullcap, lemon balm, chamomile or passion flower are excellent. Exercises such as yoga, meditation, biofeedback and other relaxation techniques are also helpful.

A perforated eardrum is a rupture to the eardrum which leaves a hole in it and results in pain and loss of hearing. It can be caused by infection, injury or loud noise. Infection of the middle ear (otitis media – see below) can result in a broken eardrum when the pressure of the swelling behind it gets too much. Pus and mucus comes out of the ear and needs to be checked for a perforated eardrum. The herbal approach is to address the infection of the middle ear (see below). A ruptured eardrum sometimes can heal by itself but in other cases, surgery may be necessary.

Earache
Glue ear (otitis media) often causes earache. Blockage of the eustachian tube (the tube that connects the middle ear to the mouth) during a cold, allergy, or upper respiratory infection and the presence of bacteria or viruses lead to the accumulation of fluid (a build-up of pus and mucus) behind the eardrum. This infection is called acute otitis media. The build up of pressurized pus in the middle ear causes earache, swelling, and redness. Since the eardrum cannot vibrate properly, it leads to hearing problems. Glue ear is particularly common in young children.

Sometimes the eardrum ruptures, and pus drains out of the ear. But more commonly, the pus and mucus remain in the middle ear due to the swollen and inflamed eustachian tube causing earache and some considerable distress especially in children.

Common symptoms of glue ear are:

- earache
- feeling of fullness or pressure

- hearing problems
- dizziness, loss of balance
- nausea, vomiting
- ear drainage
- fever

Remember, without proper treatment, damage from an ear infection can cause chronic or permanent hearing loss. Herbal treatments for earache caused by glue ear is to give effective anti-infective agents such astragalus, echinacea, garlic or goldenseal. This will combat the infection and prevent further inflammation. Other useful herbs are chamomile, licorice or mullein which will soothe the inflamed areas. The long-term strategy aims to reduce excessive catarrh which can predispose the system to middle ear infections. Herb teas containing goldenrod, hyssop, eyebright, elderflowers, marshmallow leaves or coltsfoot are all excellent choices. Dietary changes such as limiting dairy, refined sugars, simple carbohydrates, fizzy drinks and processed foods are an absolute must if further episodes are to be avoided. This will strengthen the immune system and prevent infection. Stress-busting measures are also important since stress increases the susceptibility to infection by reducing the body's resistance to it. Supplements of vitamin C and zinc may be useful in the short-term for those who frequently get ear infections as this is a sign of chronic immune deficiency. Together with herbal immune boosters, this should be sufficient to combat further infections more naturally.

Eczema

Eczema is a dry skin condition characterised by patches of inflamed, red, itchy skin. There are small fluid-filled blisters which develop and subsequently burst giving the characteristic 'weepy' skin appearance. The patches then crust over. Recurrent attacks lead to scarring and thickening of the skin which changes the colour and appearance of the skin, affecting its integrity and purpose. Severe eczema is very distressing particularly if the face, neck and hands are affected. Many children outgrow this condition and in some it is also accompanied by hay fever and/or asthma as all 3 conditions fall in the band of allergic conditions called atopic allergy.

The herbal approach is to use a range of anti-inflammatories, demulcents and skin restoratives. In this respect, herbs such as calendula cream, chamomile cream or licorice cream are excellent. Skin restoratives such as centella fixed oil or comfrey cream are great choices. Anti-pruritic creams such as chickweed will prevent the intense itching and will also soothe the skin. Long-term use of topical creams combined in a mixture that includes all these actions will restore skin integrity so that it begins to resemble healthy skin again. Internal mixtures (either tinctures and/teas) that include chamomile, centella, licorice can also be considered. A good combination for most dry skin conditions is a mixture of sarsaparilla and mahonia. As eczema is an immune condition, a herb such as echinacea is invariably added in order to modify immune responses so that inflammation is kept to a minimum in predisposed individuals.

Owing to the general dryness in the system and the lack of moisture, supplementation of hemp seed oil is highly recommended. This nutrient replenishes the fats that are essential to diet and general nutritional status. Most dry conditions occur in systems that are deficient in these essential fatty acids (notably the omega fatty acids). They are also found naturally occurring in fatty fish (such as salmon, tuna, mackerel, herring, trout & sardines) as well as some nuts (eg. walnuts) and seeds (linseeds, hemp seed and others). It is vital for the skin to have these fats for its healthy state and function. It can be added to smoothies but choose those that are not yoghurt-based as dairy aggravates the condition.

Other supplements such as vitamin C (for wound healing and for general health and vitality of the skin), as well as zinc are also highly recommended. This mineral is an essential part of our immune system and is required to modulate the immune responses in the body. Inflammatory conditions can often result from a deficiency of zinc in the diet and studies have shown it to have a beneficial effect in eczema.

General dietary & lifestyle recommendations in eczema:

- Increase fatty fish intake (good examples are listed above)
- Increase flaxseeds/linseeds. These can be bought from most supermarkets and can be easily sprinkled on top of cereals for a crunchy texture. This is high in the omega fatty acids so it is a good nutrient. Another suitable choice is hemp seed oil (as above)
- Limit all dairy intake especially cheese, milk, eggs, yoghurt etc…
- Try goat's cheese as an alternative to dairy cheese
- Limit or avoid altogether all junk food – far too many additives and chemicals that could trigger an inflammatory response in sensitive systems
- Reduce red meat where possible and eat more fatty fish & chicken instead
- Increase intake of fresh fruit and vegetables. Go organic & non-GMO whenever possible and go for variety. This will ensure you cover all bases where nutrition is concerned
- Try gluten-free foods – there could be a possible wheat sensitivity
- Plan the weekly food shopping by making a list and spend time thinking about meals way ahead so you have some control over diet and culprit foods
- Limit eating out where possible but once in a while is OK or choose foods that are 'safe' (non-culprits foods) on the menu
- Avoid wool and nylon materials in clothing
- Avoid coconut oil, lanolin and coal tar products in all toiletries
- Try almond or olive oil with a few drops of chamomile essential oil (EO) or lemon balm EO as an alternative moisturiser to the skin
- Vitamin E cream or oil is also a good moisturiser for the skin
- Sea salt baths once a week. Or add oatmeal to baths – great for nourishing the skin and an excellent moisturiser for eczema.
- Take regular exercise to boost circulation and the healing process. Exercise will also boost immunity and general health & vitality.

- Consider stress-reduction measures and relaxation techniques. Stress contributes significantly to the condition and can make an existing episode much worse.

Endometriosis

Endometriosis is a complex and debilitating disease that can affect any woman. It is a chronic and progressive condition characterised by acute episodes. It is one of the commonest benign gynaecological conditions in which tissue that would normally grow only in the endometrium (inner lining of the uterus), is found elsewhere in the abdominal and pelvic cavities, accompanied by cyclical bleeding of these tissues and the formation of painful cysts. Subsequent rupture of cysts and the resultant inflammatory process often leads to the formation of multiple adhesions. In more severe cases, endometrial tissue can migrate to other parts of the body and this presents a complicated clinical picture, particularly if there are other systems involved.

<u>Summary of herbs commonly indicated in the symptomatic approach to endometriosis</u>

Symptom	Phytochemical properties/ Pharmacological actions	Herbs of Choice
Chronic abdominal or pelvic pain	<ul><li>pelvic tonic & astringent</li><li>anti-inflammatory</li><li>analgesic</li><li>antispasmodic</li></ul>	life root cramp bark chamomile Jamaica dogwood
Ovulation pain (pain mid-cycle)	<ul><li>hormone balancer</li><li>ovarian tonic</li></ul>	pulsatilla false unicorn root chaste berry
Painful periods	<ul><li>antispasmodic</li><li>analgesic</li><li>anti-inflammatory</li></ul>	cramp bark black cohosh pulsatilla
Heavy periods	<ul><li>anti-haemorrhagic</li><li>astringent</li></ul>	yarrow beth root squaw vine
Menstrual irregularities	<ul><li>hormone balancer (oestrogenic or progesteronal)</li></ul>	chaste berry wild yam sarsaparilla
Pain on intercourse	<ul><li>anti-inflammatory</li><li>analgesic</li></ul>	pulsatilla
Pain on passing urine	<ul><li>astringent</li><li>demulcent</li><li>anti-inflammatory</li></ul>	shepherd's purse slippery elm cornsilk
Pain on bowel movement	<ul><li>anti-inflammatory</li><li>astringent</li></ul>	yarrow witch hazel
Aggravated PMS	<ul><li>hormone balancer (oestrogenic or progesteronal)</li></ul>	chaste berry milk thistle Chinese angelica
Pelvic congestion	<ul><li>decongestants</li><li>circulatory stimulants</li><li>uterine tonics</li></ul>	ginger false unicorn root yarrow

By far the most important adjunct in the management of endometriosis is addressing nutrition, since dietary factors have been shown on many occasions to be very closely linked to health. Hormonal imbalances in endometriosis can be addressed on a nutritional level and controlling oestrogen is essentially a nutritional process.

Infertility and pain are two major symptoms that can be effectively addressed through diet; certain nutrients possess pain relieving and anti-inflammatory properties which correspond to conventional medicines without the side effects. Essential fatty acids such as fish oils, evening primrose oil (EPO), starflower oil, borage oil and linseed oils are important as is Vitamin B_6 which encourages the production of progesterone and this helps rebalance the 2 main sex hormones. Other supplementary nutrients that are suggested have been summarised below.

<u>Selected nutrients of value and relevance in addressing manifestations of endometriosis</u>

NUTRIENT/FOOD ADDITIVE	COMMENT
Vitamin C	• reduces inflammation
B complex	• anti-inflammatory, analgesic and hormone balancer
Magnesium deficiency	• causes muscle cramping in abdomen & joint pains (Magnesium acts on nerves that influence the relaxation of muscles & reduce the cramping pains during menstruation)
Dioxin (pesticide)	• thought to cause immune system damage and endometriosis through its build up in fat cells
Phytooestrogens	• weak oestrogenic effect (good at reducing symptoms) • broccoli, French beans, pomegranates & fish oils encourages production of oestrogens in the body

The psychological wellbeing has equal emphasis in herbal management as is dealing with the physical symptoms. Effective herbal treatments using a range of nervines to address the psychological and emotional aspects of endometriosis remains an essential component of the management approach. Herbs such as skullcap, vervain and wood betony are all considered. A consultation with a herbalist is highly recommended in order to work out the best prescription options for each case.

ENT (Ear, Nose & Throat) problems

Common ENT problems include sinusitis, catarrh, earache, ear wax, nasal allergy and laryngitis (sore throat). Ear problems have been discussed earlier. Sinusitis is an inflammation of the sinus membranes caused invariably by an infection (usually bacterial but it can be caused by other agents that produce an inflammation of the sinus membranes) Sinuses are bone cavities which are located at various places in the face and forehead. Proper drainage of the sinuses is essential for keeping the head clear of mucus and secretions from the nasal passages. The herbal approach to treatment is firstly to consider whether the problem is acute or chronic. In acute cases, there has usually been a respiratory infection and lasts for less than a month. In chronic cases, there is some allergic response, pollutants, allergens, dust, infection or environmental factors. Anti-infective agents such as steam inhalations of myrrh oil, eucalyptus oil or clove oil are all helpful in easing breathing. However, they are also potent antimicrobials so they will combat any infection in the localised area.

Immune boosters of astragalus, wild indigo, echinacea, ginger and goldenseal are usually given as a mixture, preferable as a tea but tinctures are equally good and usually more convenient for patients. The headaches can be symptomatically treated using feverfew or meadowsweet. Chronic conditions require the same strategy as for allergies and in reviving an overburdened immune system.

Laryngitis is essentially a sore throat (inflammation of the larynx). Infective causes accompanied by symptoms of a cold requires the same approach as dealing with a cold although topical soothing agents such as syrups of thyme, licorice or wild cherry will all help. A gargle or mouthwash made from diluted tinctures of sage, chamomile, tormentil, agrimony and myrrh offers significant symptomatic relief.

Catarrh has been discussed separately.

Erectile Dysfunction (see under Impotence and Sexual Dysfunction)

Eye disorders (eg. macular degeneration, conjunctivitis, red eye, eye strain, stye)
Macular degeneration occurs mainly in the elderly and is characterised by failing eyesight particularly in fine focus and visual acuity. It may lead to blindness in time and although there are effective conventional drugs that can improve eyesight, there is no overall cure for this condition. There are a number of risk factors in macular degeneration such as smoking, a high fat diet, exposure to sunlight, ageing, high blood pressure, family history (genetic factors) and heart disease amongst others.

Herbal treatments aim to improve the blood flow in the fine capillaries that supply the retina and surrounding regions. Herbs such as ginkgo and bilberry are excellent choices in this regard. Dietary and lifestyle advice aims to address some of the underlying causes such as heart disease and high blood pressure. In some instances, a combination of high-dose beta-carotene (vitamin A), vitamin C, vitamin E, and zinc can reduce the risk of developing advanced age-related macular degeneration by about 25 percent in those patients who have earlier but significant forms of the disease.

Conjunctivitis is an inflammation of the conjunctiva, the outermost membrane of the eye and inner surface of the eyelids. It is commonly due to a bacterial or viral infection but it can also be due to allergy or environmental pollutants. It is sometimes referred to as 'red eye'. Another similar condition is blepharitis which is an inflammation of the eyelids. The herbal approach in both conditions is to address the infective state with effective eyewashes made from tea/infusions of eyebright, chamomile, dilute witch hazel, and marigold. Persistent conjunctivitis or blepharitis requires a radical look at the immune system and toxic challenge within the system and stress. Depuratives such as blue flag, poke root or cleavers will remove these toxins, combined with a good liver herb such as dandelion which will boost liver health and protect the system from foreign attack. Immune boosters such as the ginsengs (Siberian and Korean) and echinacea will improve overall resistance to infection but this needs to be supported by proper dietary and lifestyle modifications as well as practical measures to avoid or limit exposure to environmental pollutants (eg. dusty or smoky environments) and address possible allergies. Personal hygiene also needs to be looked at.

A stye is an inflammation of the sebaceous glands at the base of the eyelashes. It is usually quite visible and sometimes painful. Causes are usually infective (bacterial) but it can be brought on by stress and poor skin hygiene. Hot or warm compresses can help assisted by internal mixtures of goldenseal, echinacea and garlic to boost general immunity in order to prevent further attack. Topical eye baths (as for conjunctivitis) will also provide symptomatic relief. Persistent styes requires removal of the toxic challenge so herbs such as blue flag may be used but a herbalist will be able to work out the best long-term prescription that includes modifications to diet, lifestyle and skin hygiene measures to tackle the problem for good.

Eye strain can be caused by a number of factors such as poor light, eyesight problems, computer glare and over use of the eye muscles from long distance to near distance focusing. Symptoms can be headache, poor concentration, blurred vision and sore eye muscles, dry, irritated or watery eyes. Twitching of the eye muscles can also occur which is indicative of eye strain and general fatigue. Apart from identifying the cause of the eyestrain, practical measures to limit or avoid the cause is always advised. Soothing tired eyes through herbal eye washes containing infusions of chamomile, marigold, witch hazel or eyebright will help. Stress-busting measures will help alleviate some of the headaches and sore neck muscles that may also be the root cause of the headache. Physical exercise is also advised as it gives a host of benefits and will provide a balance to whatever activity is the cause of the eyestrain. Other measures such as herb teas containing lemon balm, chamomile and/or passion flower will help soothe and calm frazzled nerves. If long hours in front of the computer screen are unavoidable, then placing a plant (or two) near it to soak up the radiation will limit some of the exposure. Regular breaks is a must and doing something very different out of work hours is an absolute necessity as are appropriate relaxation techniques, such as listening to music, meditation and exercise.

F

Fibroids
Fibroids are growths of muscle tissue that occur in the womb (uterus). They are not cancerous (that is they are benign) and can be easily treated. It occurs in about 20-50% of women and usually in the age group of 30-40s shrinking in size after the menopause. The size of these fibroids can vary from the size of a pea to a size of a melon. The most common symptoms are very heavy menstrual bleeding, abdominal pain, changes in bowel function, changes in bladder function and in some cases, infertility.

The exact causes of fibroids are unclear although it does seem to be dependent on the female hormone oestrogen. This may partly explain why they spontaneously shrink after the menopause because the ovaries stop producing this hormone at this time of life.

In some cases, the fibroids can spread to other parts of the body causing complications and immense distress to patients. The herbal approach to treating fibroids is firstly to ascertain the extent of the growth, the severity of the symptoms and to address possible complications. Further, any impact on fertility will also have to be discussed with the patient.

Some of the traditional remedies include yarrow as this is great for improving blood flow to the pelvic region. Antispasmodics such as cramp bark or chamomile are great for relieving pain caused by muscular cramps. In cases of very heavy bleeding, anti-haemorrhagic herbs such as shepherd's purse or lady's mantle prove useful. A nice tea that patients quite like is a combination of all of the above herbs plus nettle or ginger as additional herbs. The tea needs to be drunk several times during the periods and 2 or 3 cups a day before it starts.

The main herb for reducing or shrinking the size of any fibroid is the tree of life (*thuja* or *arbor vitae*). It is also used for shrinking a number of other growths in the body such as warts and polyps, as well as cancerous growths. Hormonal balancers are also required as this is very much an oestrogen-dependent condition. Herbs such as wild yam, chaste berry and false unicorn root are usually considered by herbalists.

Nervines are also a good idea as the nervous system needs to be supported, particularly in a vulnerable patient. Herbs such as chamomile, vervain, skullcap or the ginsengs would be good choices. Supplements of iron are also suggested due to the heavy blood loss and to prevent iron-deficiency anaemia. Herb teas containing gentian and nettle will also address this. The ginsengs will also boost general energy levels and vitality. Nutritional aspects should be carefully considered too and although a healthy diet may not reduce the fibroids, it may help reduce some of the symptoms. Other measures include:

- avoiding alcohol, sugar, refined foods and saturated fats. They make it difficult for the body to regulate hormones. This can increase cramps and bloating. Switch to whole foods, grains and pulses.
- increasing intake of fresh fruits and vegetables, particularly broccoli and spinach – they may also help the body regulate its oestrogen levels.
- Ensuring plenty of vitamin B intake, calcium, magnesium and potassium – these nutrients will help reduce cramps and bloating.

In diagnosed cases, it is best to seek a consultation with a herbalist rather than self-medicating in order to have a thorough assessment of the condition and so that treatment is tailor-made. This will be more effective in the long-term as underlying causes can be properly addressed and the focus on 'treating the patient, rather than the condition' can have greater clinical benefits than merely treating the symptoms.

Fibromyalgia

Fibromyalgia is an increasingly common problem characterised by diffuse joint, muscle or bone pain and accompanied by fatigue. Some healthcare practitioners also refer to this as fibrositis. Many experts think that fibromyalgia is the same as chronic fatigue syndrome (CFS), or at least variations of the same because both present with pain and fatigue. Sleep and mental function is disturbed and the trigger can often be traced to an injury, or physical or emotional trauma. There are also abnormal levels of several chemicals, such as serotonin and substance P; these are used in the body to transmit and respond to pain signals. Many doctors believe fibromyalgia to be a psychological or psychiatric disorder because there is a distinct absence of biological markers for the condition and this proves additionally frustrating for patients.

The herbal treatment approach is quite complex due to the very complexity of the problem. However, the main aim is to address pain, reduce inflammation, stimulate certain hormones and modulate immune responses. Nervines are also useful in tackling the emotional aspects of the condition such as depression, stress effects and a certain listlessness that often accompanies the condition. In this respect, St. John's Wort is useful both externally (oil can be used in muscle rubs) and internally to treat any feelings of depression.

Siberian ginseng is an energizing herb that can help resolve the fatigue associated with fibromyalgia. A reputable brand of the standardized extract can be taken as a supplement. Other notable herbs that are used include turmeric, passion flower, valerian and cramp bark (for pain and inflammation), echinacea, cayenne and goldenseal (for boosting immunity) and ginkgo for improving circulation to the muscles and improving mental function. For joint symptoms, devil's claw is good as it is both anti-inflammatory and an effective pain reliever. Skullcap and valerian will improve sleep and licorice will support the adrenal glands. These produce cortisol which are the body's natural corticosteroid and an effective anti-inflammatory.

A full consultation with a herbalist is required in order to fully assess the condition and to specify treatments in each case. Nutritional supplements and changes to diet may also be recommended.

Flu

This is short for influenza. See under influenza.

Frozen shoulder

Frozen shoulder (adhesive capsulitis) is a disorder characterized by pain and stiffness or loss of mobility in the shoulder. The process involves hardening and subsequent shrinking of the surrounding shoulder joint. This results in the loss of movement and joint stiffness. It can be diagnosed by x-ray, an examination by the doctor or an MRI (magnetic resonance imaging) scan. Causes of frozen shoulder can be varied from injury to diabetes and thyroid disorders.

The herbal treatment approach is to use a combination of topical creams, sometimes in combination with conventional treatments and manual exercises to slowly improve mobility of the joint. Topical creams can contain anti-inflammatories, pain relievers and circulatory stimulants. Herbs such as white willow, meadowsweet, devil's claw, cayenne, wintergreen and prickly ash are all excellent choices. A consultation with a herbalist is advised so that the best combination of herbs can be specifically chosen as well as the best methods of administration, particularly if conventional drugs are being prescribed.

Fungal infections (*Tinea corporis & Tinea pedis*)

Fungal infections are common but pose a potentially serious problem if left untreated. The most common fungal infections are athlete's foot and candidiasis (thrush). These have been previously described. Effective anti-fungal herbs are calendula (marigold), tree of life (*arbor vitae*), poke root and tea tree oil.

119

G

Gall bladder problems

The gall bladder is an important organ which stores and secretes bile, a substance than helps in the breakdown of fats. Many waste products, including a blood pigment is secreted into bile which is later excreted from the body. Problems with the gall bladder can happen in 2 ways. There could be an insufficiency in bile production from the liver or a blockage in its secretion into the gut. Both problems result in poor digestive function, particularly the fats. Symptoms include nausea, a feeling of fullness, pain in the abdominal region and an intolerance to fat or fatty meals. Herbs that improve gall bladder function include artichoke, fringe tree bark and fumitory. Bile production from the liver is improved by dandelion, barberry, fringe tree bark, wormwood and milk thistle.

Another problem of the gall bladder is stones which require emergency treatment in severe cases; the pain can be intractable (biliary colic). Gall stones can be cholesterol-based or developed from bile pigment, or indeed both as is usually the case. The bigger the size of the stone, the greater the risk of blockage in narrow cavities, tubes and ducts. Any herb that encourages the free flow of bile will help disperse the stone so long as it is not already in the bile duct (in which case, herbs can make it worse by blocking the flow of bile, upset the digestion of fats and cause inflammation, infection and even jaundice). Any herbs that increase the production and flow of bile will encourage gallstones to move along. The best use for herbs is for preventing gallbladder attacks in the first place. Oregon grape root (mahonia), fringe tree bark, milk thistle and turmeric all help prevent gallstones by making bile less saturated. Inflammation can be reduced by chamomile and cramp bark to help prevent painful spasms. A diet that contains too much refined food and too little fibre may at least be partially responsible for gallstones. With such a diet, the gallbladder secretes less acid into the bile fluid. The body needs this acid to dissolve cholesterol. Without sufficient acid, cholesterol builds up into stones. It is highly recommended that conventional treatment is sought in the first instance and thereafter, it is a matter of redressing digestive, liver and gall bladder function. Dietary changes have to include the cutting down of fatty meals, refined foods, processed meals and alcohol.

Gastric reflux

This is sometimes simply referred to as acid reflux or heartburn, meaning the backward flow of food from the stomach or gullet back into the mouth. Symptoms include acid indigestion, nausea, vomiting and difficulty in swallowing. It is usually caused by the loss of muscle control in the region that regulates the entry of food into the stomach, probably caused by drugs such as antacids and aspirin.

The herbal approach is to address the underlying cause which looks at the strength and tone of the muscle in question. Addressing the symptoms such as inflammation and burning sensation caused by the acid involves using demulcents and anti-inflammatories such as chamomile, marshmallow or slippery elm. Other useful herbs include licorice and comfrey but in some cases surgery may be necessary to restore the control of the sphincter muscle. Dietary changes involve switching to a bland diet, avoiding spicy and peppery foods, cutting out alcohol and ensuring a low salt, low fibre diet.

Gastritis

Gastritis is a general term used to describe the inflammation of the stomach lining, it can be acute or chronic. Causes of the condition can be varied such as infection, stomach acid, nutritional deficiencies, smoking, medication, stress or alcohol amongst others. Symptoms include nausea, vomiting, abdominal pain and a loss of appetite.

Before administering any herbal treatments, the cause is usually identified and any other factors that could be making the symptoms worse. Infective causes require antimicrobials such as goldenseal or garlic. Nutritional deficiencies require dietary changes after initial supplementation of the required nutrient (usually it is a vitamin or mineral deficiency). Other dietary causes require the same approach. Stress reduction measures are also useful as are herbs that reduce inflammation and soothe irritated linings. Herbs such as slippery elm, marshmallow, chamomile, meadowsweet and cinnamon are good choices for symptomatic relief. A consultation with a herbalist is advised so that an individual prescription can be decided, especially in chronic cases.

Gastroentritis

Gastroenteritis is a severe form of food poisoning producing vomiting and diarrhoea. It is caused by an infective agent (can be bacterial, viral or parasitic). It causes inflammation of the stomach and although in some cases, the condition will resolve itself, care needs to be taken in order to prevent dehydration especially in severe cases. The condition is highly infectious so care needs to be taken regarding food and personal hygiene; it is also best to stay away from work or school.

Herbal treatments include antimicrobials (for infective causes) such as garlic, astragalus and golden seal. Anti-inflammatories such as chamomile and licorice are recommended as well as astringents such as agrimony, and demulcents such as marshmallow or slippery elm to soothe the inflamed and irritated lining. Additionally, a good liver herb such as milk thistle or schizandra is also recommended to boost liver health and to improve digestive function after the debility. A consultation with a herbalist is highly recommended so that other factors can be considered and to devise a long-term strategy to improve immunity in order to prevent recurrence.

Gingivitis

Gingivitis is an inflammation of the gums caused by poor dental hygiene, poorly fitted dental material (eg. fillings, dentures) a build up of plaque and bacterial infection. Preventative measures should address all of the above causes. However, the condition could also happen in diabetes, pregnancy, vitamin C deficiency and malnutrition amongst others. Herbal mouthwashes deal with the symptoms but other measures are necessary to treat the underlying cause in other cases. A combination of the following herbs makes a good mouthwash: a tea or diluted tincture of sage, witch hazel, myrrh, chamomile, tormentil and agrimony. Supplements of vitamin C in cases of deficiency (signs of scurvy) is required as well as good dental hygiene and dietary changes in other cases (eg. low sugar diet in diabetes).

Glaucoma

Glaucoma is a condition of the eyes characterised by impaired vision which can eventually lead to blindness. It is caused by a build up of pressure from the fluid in the eyeballs that press onto the lens, thus distorting the vision. Fluid build up is usually a feature of other conditions, notably high blood pressure so treatment usually involves measures to reduce this. Other common causes are diabetes, stress, medication, injury and family history.

Treatment of the underlying cause is the first step. These will be specific to the cause. General herbs for vision include bilberry, ginkgo, calendula and elder berries (increases vascular integrity and circulation). Buckwheat is another excellent choice as this contains noticeable quantities of rutin, an important bioflavonoid. Supplements of vitamins A and C, beta carotene and magnesium and also advised.

Gout

This condition is characterised by pain, swelling, redness and heat in the joints, classically in the big toe although any joint can be affected. It is caused by an abnormality of uric acid which results in crystals of them being deposited within the body, notably in the joint cartilages. In severe cases, the deposits increase in size and burst through the skin discharging the uric acid in the process. A common complication of the condition is kidney stones which are caused by the increased levels of uric acid in the blood. Pain and loss of mobility are 2 characteristics of this condition.

Gout is a metabolic disorder and it is the case that either too much uric acid is being produced (diet-induced or enzyme deficiency) or that the kidneys do not excrete enough of it. It is inconclusive whether poor diet and lifestyle or a genetic predisposition is to blame. However, part of the treatment involves a low intake of purines (a type of amino acid found in protein rich foods such as red meats and some fish), low alcohol intake (especially beer) and switching to vegetable protein and increasing fruit intake especially the red berries (eg. cherries and strawberries). Additionally, fresh vegetables, diluted celery juice, distilled water, vitamin B-complex and vitamin C can all help lower uric acid in the blood. It is important to maintain a healthy weight as obesity is a risk factor.

Herbal treatments are really for addressing some of the symptoms in addition to making radical changes to the diet. In a similar manner to arthitis, anti-inflammatories and analgesics are highly favoured (see under arthritis). However, some of the herbal diuretics such as dandelion leaf, boldo leaf and celery seeds exert effective anti-arthritic properties. Another herb of choice for gout is nettle tea as this will lower uric acid levels in the blood. However, chronic cases require conventional treatments with more powerful anti-inflammatories such as steroid injections or non-steroidal anti-inflammatory drugs.

H

Haemorrhoids (piles)

Haemorrhoids are also commonly known as piles. They are swollen blood vessels in the rectum and anus that enlarge to form lumps called piles. In some cases, these lumps burst when the bowels are opened causing blood to leak out through the anus. Piles are usually a feature of constipation. Blood in the stools is never normal so other conditions of the bowel should also be investigated to rule out more serious disorders (such as inflammatory bowel disease or cancer). Other symptoms of piles include pain and discomfort in the lower bowels as well as itching around the anus.

Herbal treatment of piles always considers aspects of diet and making necessary changes especially in increasing the amount of fibre in the diet. Foods that are naturally high in fibre are fruits and vegetables as well as wheatbran, muesli, oats, flaxseeds and psyllium husks. Avoid refined and processed foods as far as possible and eat the fruits in their whole form rather than juicing them.

Herbal creams can be applied topically to shrink external piles. Preparations containing witch hazel, oak bark, sage in a horse chestnut base cream can be used. Internally, herbal laxatives such as rhubarb root, senna or buckthorn bark may assist in bowel movement but this is a short-term measure. Effective long-term solutions only lie in changing the diet on a permanent basis.

Halitosis

This is commonly known as bad breath. Temporary bad breath may be as a result of eating strong foods with pungent odours such as garlic or onions, or even smoking. It is the chronic bad breath that is of concern and requires treatment. There can be a number of causes why bad breath occurs. It may be due to poor dental hygiene which results in bacteria colonising the mouth and causing bad breath. Some of the stronger mouth washes should address that as well as improving dental hygiene. Bad breath can also be caused by throat, mouth or stomach infections so dealing with that is a priority. Antimicrobials such as goldenseal or astragalus can be taken. Mouthwashes containing mint, fennel seeds, aniseed or dill seeds are all good. Gargles containing myrrh oil (diluted in water) will eliminate any throat infection. Poor elimination and liver health can also result in bad breath as this will be a sign of toxic overload. Depuratives such as blue flag or burdock are required as well as a liver herb such as dandelion.

Other causes can include chronic liver failure so specialist advice is necessary. In all cases of chronic bad breath, a consultation with a herbalist is needed in the first instance in order to identify the cause and to work out effective treatment strategies from dietary changes and practical measures to specific herbal medicines.

Hay fever

This is also called allergic rhinitis and much of the same treatment approaches apply as in allergies. (see under Allergies for herbal approaches).

In addition, the specific symptoms of hay fever include itchy, watery eyes, constant sneezing, sore and red eyes etc. Boosting immunity is necessary so herbs such as echinacea, marigold or ginseng will help. After this, the traditional allergy herbs such as nettle, eyebright, elderflowers, ephedra, ginkgo and chamomile will all address the various symptoms of hay fever. Supplements such as quercetin and omega 3 essential fatty acids will replenish the system with the important nutrients. Some have found that butterbur (petasites) particularly effective. However, a consultation with a herbalist is strongly advised so that an individual treatment plan can be worked out and to identify which pollens are the culprits in each case.

Headache

The underlying cause of the common headache should always be identified first before beginning treatment. Persistent headaches should always be examined more thoroughly and this may require a consultation with either a doctor or a medical herbalist to identify the root cause. It may simply be a matter of taking practical measures to eliminate the cause (which could be things such as long hours in front of the computer screen or a need to correct eyesight/ glasses prescription, infection or stress). In more serious cases, it could be a sign of dehydration, meningitis, head injury or tumours amongst others.

The common headache in its simplest form is the result of constricted blood flow to the brain. This can be due to muscular tension in the neck and shoulders, often caused by stress, anxiety or bad posture. Relieving this type of tension headache is to address the stress and anxiety and various practical measures (eg. relaxation techniques, stress-busting measures) can be taken before resorting to medicines. Relaxants such as wood betony, lemon balm, skullcap or passion flower can help. Migraines require more specific help and only the individual will really know how it manifests and what can be done to relieve it. Herbs such as wood betony, feverfew (best to eat a few of the fresh leaves as this is more effective), butterbur and ginkgo are useful. Other useful herbs are valerian, chamomile and yellow jasmine but it is strongly advisable to seek proper professional help before self-medicating as the headache could be a sign of something more serious and this needs to be ruled out before herbal treatments can be given.

Head lice

Head lice is a common problem and it usually occurs in children although it can affect any one of any age. The lice are parasites and feed on the blood by sucking it through the skin. The female lays its eggs (nits) in sacs which are glued to a hair. These take seven to ten days to hatch. The lice then take seven to fourteen days to become mature and ready to reproduce. The total numbers of lice can therefore rise very quickly. It is passed on by direct contact from one hair to another or from one head to another.

Home remedies involve removing the nits and live lice with a lice comb and/or tweezers. Herbal hair washes containing tea tree oil, Chinese wormwood and /or eucalyptus oil are all effective.

Heartburn

Heartburn is acid indigestion which is caused by gastric reflux. See above for herbal treatments for this condition.

Heavy periods

Heavy periods is a real blight on patients' lives as the consequences can be serious leading to iron-deficiency anaemia, fatigue, weakness, low blood pressure, dizziness and fainting. Sometimes the heavy bleeding can be a sign of fibroids so this will have to be investigated if needed. In other cases, it could just be that it has always been that way so patients have had a lifetime of this problem and get used to dealing with pain.

Herbal astringents such as shepherd's purse, beth root or lady's mantle are needed in any herbal prescription but also uterine tonics such as raspberry leaf or white peony to tone and strengthen the uterus with supplementation of vitamin K in cases of abnormalities in the blood clotting process. Additionally, hormone balancers such as chaste berry or false unicorn root are good choices as they will regulate any menstrual irregularity or abnormality. Supplements of iron (liquid or tablet form) may also be required to address any iron-deficiency anaemia.

Herpes (cold sores, shingles, post-herpetic neuralgia)

Cold sores have been previously discussed and this is caused by the type 1 *Herpes simplex* virus. The type 2 *Herpes simplex* virus causes genital herpes and this is a sexually transmitted disease that requires specialist treatment via the doctor, at sexual health clinics or genito-urinary medicine (GUM) clinics. The *Herpes zoster* virus causes shingles and strong anti-viral treatment is required. It occurs in those who have had chicken pox previously and symptoms include a burning, intense pain along areas of the body serviced by specific nerve pathways. Parts of the body affected are usually the ribs, back, arms, legs and the side of the face with the person experiencing lethargy, headache or fever. Topically, the lesions can be treated using herbs such as cayenne or chilli pepper, St. John's Wort oil, lemon balm, skullcap and licorice. Turmeric, mullein and aloe vera are also good choices as between them, they will tackle the pain and soothe irritated and inflamed skin patches.

The herbal approach for any *herpes* infection will generally follow the same form as cold sores but to address the various types of herpes is also important. Treatment of the underlying cause is necessary as shingles usually occurs in a weakened immune system, the periods following chronic illness. It is best to consult a herbalist to work out an individual treatment plan in each case.

High Cholesterol (Hypercholesterolaemia)

Many people in the West probably have raised cholesterol levels and there are many products that are being commercially marketed to address this problem. However, the best and most effective way of dealing with raised levels on a long-term basis is through diet and lifestyle, depending on the severity of the condition. Family history and a predisposition to raised levels of the 'bad' cholesterol has some part to play and susceptible individuals should have their levels checked as a matter of caution.

Herbs that are effective in reducing levels of cholesterol are garlic, artichoke, turmeric and a substance extracted form the myrrh tree called guggul. Guggul is a sticky resin that is more commonly used in Ayurvedic herbal medicine but it is becoming more widespread in its use because the numbers of people being diagnosed with raised cholesterol levels are increasing.

Cardiovascular exercise is also key to reducing the levels of 'bad' cholesterol whilst increasing the levels of the 'good' cholesterol. High cholesterol foods include red meats, butter, lard, fried foods, soft cheeses, avocado, eggs and foods high in refined sugars, amongst others. These should be limited as far as possible especially in the early stages of reducing cholesterol levels. It is important not to eliminate all foods as some of them will contain important nutrients but attempt to achieve a balance and moderation, combined with a healthier lifestyle. Increase intakes of fermented soy products (miso, tempeh, tamari and shoyu) and limit the amount of saturated fats and processed foods as far as possible. Switch to vegetarian alternatives as much as possible and avoid alcohol and give up smoking. A consultation with a nutritionist is a must as well as a herbalist who will devise a phased programme of how healthy levels of cholesterol can be achieved that will not compromise intake of essential nutrients from natural food sources.

Hives

Hives are raised, itchy, red patches of skin that occur from an allergic reaction from a range of substances from prescription drugs and foods to exposure to the cold. The treatment of hives follows the same protocol as for allergies in general. Please refer to this section on how herbal medicines can treat this problem. Topical creams made from chamomile, centella oil and licorice cream can soothe the skin as can aloe vera gel. A tea made from nettle, yarrow and burdock can also also help.

Hypertension
(high blood pressure) – see Blood disorders

Hyperthyroidism (overactive thyroid) – see Thyroid Disorders
The thyroid gland makes the hormones thyroxine which regulates our metabolic rate, that is, all the body's biochemical processes including how quickly energy is released from our energy stores and food in order to sustain us. The gland is under the control of higher centres in the brain so the regulation of our metabolic processes is a finely controlled process. Sometimes, things can go wrong with the gland itself or indeed the higher centres that control the thyroid. This can lead to abnormal levels of the hormone, which can be too high or too low.

The most common cause of hyperthyroidism is Grave's disease which is characterised by a goitre, an enlargement of the thyroid gland which is visible as a swelling in the neck. The symptoms of excessive levels of thyroid hormone are numerous but ostensibly it is a speeding up of all the metabolic process and the manifestation of them. These include weight loss, irritability, anxiety or restlessness, excessive sweating, insomnia, itchy skin, heat intolerance, rapid heart rate and a shortness of breath amongst many others.

The herbal approach is to attempt to regulate levels of the hormone in the first instance. The most notable herb is bugleweed (also known as gypsywort) which reduces levels of iodine of which there is too much in this condition. A tincture of the herb can be used as a supplement, mix water with 5 drops of the tincture and drink three times everyday as a herbal treatment and preventative measure. A herbalist may prescribe this as part of a symptomatic approach in dealing with some of the other problems that patients experience. Long-term strategies involve examining the immune system especially in Grave's disease as this is an autoimmune disease caused by antibodies being made against the thyroid gland, causing it to produce too much hormone. Most autoimmune disorders cause a lot of inflammation to occur in the body, an extract of turmeric called curcumin is a very effective anti-inflammatory and can deal with all disorders or inflammations brought on by such conditions.

The psychological state of the patient is also important as stress levels are increased as are symptoms of it such as anxiety and irritability. Nervines have their use in this regard so herbs such as lemon balm, skullcap or Indian ginseng with a good vitamin B complex can be very useful. Autoimmune disorders in the body are often reduced and alleviated by essential fatty acids so evening primrose oil, hemp seed oil or flaxseed oil are good choices for supplementation. Other useful supplements are vitamin C, minerals like zinc, copper and selenium, including the element essential for thyroid function: iodine along with the amino acid tyrosine can be used to promote the healthy functioning of the thyroid gland.

Hypothyroidism (underactive thyroid) – see Thyroid Disorders

An underactive thyroid gland is known as hypothyroidism and this leads to low levels of the thyroid hormone. Symptoms include fatigue, slowed speech, slow heart rate, impaired memory, depression, constipation and weight gain amongst many others. Like hyperthyroidism, this is a complex clinical picture and treatment may require conventional methods. Historically, the cause of hypothyroidism was due to an insufficiency in the mineral iodine, which is an integral constituent of the hormone itself. In the West, there is no shortage of iodine in our diets but this does not mean that people get enough from their foods, invariably because of poor choices. The herb bladderwrack, also known as kelp, is a seaweed that is sourced from marine waters and therefore contains significant quantities of iodine which addresses the shortage of iodine that occurs in hypothyroid cases. However, this needs to be taken under supervision of a herbal practitioner as sometimes patients can overload on iodine by taking supplements of it. Herbal prescriptions that combine this herb with herbs that addresses the other symptoms is usually the case. Good sources of iodine from foods are sea salt, seafood, bread, milk and cheese. However, this does not address low thyroid hormone as a result of genetic causes, radioactive therapy for an overactive thyroid or problems in the higher centres in the brain that regulate the thyroid gland (can be a pituitary gland tumour or previous surgery or treatment).

I

Impetigo

Impetigo is an infectious skin disorder caused by a bacterial infection and characterised by blisters which quickly turn to golden-green crusts. It usually occurs in children and in hot, moist climates but in colder climates it is usually an indication of poor hygiene standards. Conventional treatment is to use an antibiotic ointment. The herbal approach is to boost immunity and to combat the infection so echinacea and burdock is especially effective against the actual bacterium that causes impetigo. Cleavers or poke root can be used to support the lymphatic system to clear the bacteria. These may be given in the form of tinctures or teas. The oil of myrrh is particular good topically as it is antibacterial (1 drop twice a day). Also, tea tree oil can be applied to the affected areas using a mixture of 3 drops of the essential oil for each teaspoon of water, and lightly cleanse the affected area.

A fresh clove of garlic, an antibiotic, can be crushed, mixed with honey and taken three times a day.

Dietary recommendations would be to cut out dairy foods (could try goat's milk and/or cheese), cut out all refined foods and switch to whole foods, eliminate all processed foods with lots of additives, preservatives, colourings and foods containing refined flour.

Impotence (also look under Sexual Dysfunction)

Impotence is also referred to as erectile dysfunction (ED). It occurs when a man has difficulty with either getting an erection or with keeping an erection for long enough to allow satisfactory sexual activity. It is one of the most common sexual problems and affects around half of all men over 40 at some point. It becomes more common and severe as men get older. However, only a fraction of affected men seek help.

There are a number of causes of ED. In around two thirds of cases, there are physical problems affecting the blood supply. However, there is a complex relationship between physical and psychological aspects of sexual function. Additionally lifestyle factors such as drinking too much alcohol, medicines and diet can all be causes of ED.

The treatment of ED depends very much on the cause if it can be identified. Factors that can be influenced such as diet and lifestyle changes will be advised. Herbs that are reputed to have a tonic effect on the male reproductive organs such as Korean ginseng and sarsaparilla may be given by a herbalist. Other notable herbs may include damiana but there is no single herb that is prescribed specifically for ED as it is very much a complex case. Emotional health and the psychological well-being of the patient is closely examined and any impact of stress is duly addressed through appropriate nervines. Some of the traditional herbal medicines for ED have been more recently considered, particularly in light of the fact that Viagra® does not work for all patients, and some have reported extreme adverse effects. Herbs such as the yohimbe bark, extracts from the muira puama plant, an extract from the makandi plant and yellow vine (also known as caltrop or puncture vine) is a herb more commonly used within ayurvedic medicine and in Chinese herbal medicine, the horney goat weed is popularly used to promote sexual activity and to treat impotence. It is strongly recommended a diagnosis from your doctor and then a consultation with a herbalist to work out the best herbal treatments for ED. Emotional or psychological causes need appropriate therapy from relevant specialists.

Indigestion

Almost everyone has experienced a bout of indigestion. This is characterised by nausea or a feeling of fullness following a heavy meal that is difficult to digest. More serious causes of indigestion can include acid indigestion (or gastric reflux – see above), peptic or duodenal ulcers, pancreatitis, gall bladder problems. All these require a visit to the doctor especially if there is pain as well. Indigestion can also be a part of morning sickness during pregnancy.

Simple cases of indigestion require a close examination of diet and lifestyle. Poor eating habits and poor choices of food can all trigger indigestion. Equally food intolerances, now a huge part of gut symptoms are becoming increasingly common. A food intolerance test is strongly advised in that case. A clinical nutritionist, should be able to perform this easily or a referral to a hospital dietician from your doctor can be organised.

Herbal treatments are specific to the cause of the indigestion. Acid reflux has already been discussed but using demulcents and anti-inflammatories such as chamomile, marshmallow or slippery elm have a general purpose in reducing the burning sensation and feelings of nausea. Other useful herbs include licorice and comfrey leaf and specific anti-nausea herbs such as ginger or black horehound. Dietary changes involve switching to a bland diet, avoiding spicy and peppery foods, cutting out alcohol and ensuring a low salt, low fibre diet. The more serious causes require a definitive diagnosis and a management of the condition through proper diet, lifestyle and herbal medicines.

Infertility

There is no question that infertility in the UK is on the increase with a predicted incidence of 1 in 3 within the next 10 years. That is an alarming trend. However, some of this trend can be explained in that women are having babies later in life, environmental oestrogens reducing the sperm count in men, obesity, stress, increase in the numbers of female reproductive disorders, poor nutritional habits that compromise reproductive function, increased incidence of cancers etc…

The causes must be correctly identified and treated wherever possible and that includes an assessment of male fertility (sperm numbers, motility and shape). Herbs can do very little unless there is an established hormonal link or imbalance in diagnosed cases. Correcting problems such as menstrual irregularities, polycystic ovaries, endometriosis or fibroids through herbal medicines can improve fertility dramatically. A consultation with a herbalist is highly recommended if there are problems in conceiving. If there is a functional disorder then this must be corrected first and this can be achieved naturally through herbal supplements where possible before conventional treatments. A good nutritional supplement should include a multivitamin and mineral supplement, folic acid, vitamin B_{12}, zinc, selenium and the essential fatty acids. A healthy, balanced, natural and wholefood diet is essential as are lifestyle changes such as quitting smoking, reducing weight if obese or overweight, cutting down alcohol and stimulants such as coffee and tea, reducing pollution as much as possible especially from pesticide residues and plastics. Switch to organic foods where possible. Importantly, the frequency of intercourse is also a significantly influential factor in fertility and can simply be increased by having sex more frequently especially around the time of ovulation. Also, not thinking about having babies is necessary as is making the association of making love with making a baby; a pattern of thinking that places a huge burden and anxiety on both parties. Additionally, stress hormones can adversely impact on fertility quite significantly.

Inflammatory Bowel Disease or **IBD** (Crohn's Disease & Ulcerative Colitis)

Crohn's disease has previously been discussed (see above). Ulcerative colitis (UC) is the other inflammatory bowel disease that has a very similar appearance and symptoms to Crohn's and often doctors find it difficult to distinguish between the two because of these similarities. UC however, tends to affect more women than men and it is characterised by an inflamed, swollen and extensively ulcerated colon (lower intestine). The bowel may become dangerously thinned through persistent ulcerations and may perforate causing complications and severe pain. There are recurrent bouts of diarrhoea containing blood, mucus and pus in the stools. The condition can predispose the individual to cancer so regular check ups are necessary. Surgical removal of affected parts of the bowel may sometimes be necessary. It is a very distressing condition for patients made worse by the fact that conventional treatment involves long term use of steroid drugs given by mouth, as suppositories or as enemas.

Herbal medicine focuses on two aspects: the psychological well-being of the patient and in managing the symptoms. Many of the herbs that are used in Crohn's also serve well in UC. Therefore herbs such as chamomile, marshmallow and comfrey leaf are good for reducing inflammation and initiating healing of the mucous membrane linings of the gut. Fenugreek, tormentil and goldenseal are good choices too. Modulating immune responses are important so immune herbs such as echinacea are useful and due to the long-term steroid treatment, patients are usually adrenally suppressed so good herbs such as licorice or borage to support this organ is also advised. Strict dietary restrictions are imposed such as a high carbohydrate diet which is bland is specifically recommended. A varied diet of meat, fish, eggs, poultry, most vegetables, nuts and some fruits and sugars is also particularly useful. Supplements of vitamins, minerals and probiotics can be helpful because the nutritional status of the patient can be severely compromised but it is best to seek advice from a herbalist or a clinical nutritionist because certain supplements can make UC worse.

Inflammatory disorders

Inflammatory disorders can range from allergy to arthritis, from cancer to heart attack and diabetes. The list is quite extensive and almost every human condition has some association with inflammation. This is particularly true in the elderly because the immune system becomes weakened with age and the responses become modified or even inappropriate. This is particularly true of some of the autoimmune diseases. There is very little that herbal medicine can do with some of the more serious medical conditions that require conventional medicines and urgent medical attention. However, boosting immune responses or modulating them can be of benefit in some cases. Herbs such as the ginsengs, wild indigo, astragalus, garlic or goldenseal will strengthen the immune system and make it more robust against future attack. Modulating the immune system, especially in cases of autoimmunity or indeed allergy with echinacea is also essential. Examining the lymphatic system is also important as this contains some of our secondary immune cells. They play a vital role in defence and disperse accumulation of lymph fluid, preventing them from causing congestion so their health is very important. Good lymphatic herbs are marigold, poke root and blue flag (amongst many others).

Reducing the toxic load on the system is key, because this will eliminate the trigger for the inflammation so the detoxifying role of the liver must be boosted. Good liver herbs are dandelion, milk thistle, Chinese magnolia vine and fringe tree. In general, supplements of vitamin C and zinc are usually recommended for general immune health.

Influenza

This is a viral infection caused by the influenza virus, often referred to as the 'flu' and giving symptoms similar to the common cold. Unlike the common cold however, there is usually a fever, severe headache and more extensive muscle fatigue that can leave the patient quite debilitated. In the immune compromised individual, the flu can be a serious condition and can require urgent medical attention. This is particularly true of the elderly and very young children.

The herbal approach to treating the flu is a more advanced case of treating the cold so stronger doses of key herbs are used (ginseng, astragalus, echinacea and goldenseal). Herbal teas that address the fever are very useful as patients have often lost their appetite and constant fevers may have caused them to lose fluid. Herb teas containing elderflowers, yarrow and mint are all great. They will also be useful in the common cold.

Bedrest and plenty of fluids are essential, gradually introducing nutritious broths and soups. The long-term strategy is to improve immunity through herbal supplementation in the initial stages but it is better to achieve this through a proper diet that makes the system more robust. A consultation with a herbalist is advised to work out a treatment and diet plan that can boost immunity and general health to prevent further attack from the influenza virus.

Insomnia

An inability to fall asleep or having an interrupted sleep is one of the most irritating conditions that can cause severe disruption to a person's life. The short and long term consequences can be devastating to not only the patient's quality of life but also on their physical, mental and psychological health & well-being. The benefits of sleep have been highlighted elsewhere (Chapter 1 and Chapter 5). The causes of insomnia can vary from the psychological and emotional disturbances to simple biological and physical ones.

The causes have to examined thoroughly before treatment can begin because underlying causes must be addressed if the insomnia is to be successfully treated. In cases of psychological distress, there is great benefit from counselling or psychotherapy. Similarly, a range of other therapies for relaxing the body can also be beneficial so a relaxing bath, a sauna or a session in the steam room would be ideal. Strange as it may sound, exercise is great for sleep because it will make the body tired and this will assist in falling asleep. Sometimes, the excess energy that builds up through a lack of exercise and physical activity can make the body more alert at night time which will not help in falling asleep. Similarly, an active mind will also not help sleep so relaxation techniques, meditation, rest and learning to 'switch off' are vital to sleep.

Herbal relaxants, sedatives and the stronger hypnotics are used in conjunction with lifestyle changes and perhaps dietary changes in some cases. Herbs of choice are valerian, hops, passion flower, lemon balm, Californian poppy, chamomile, Jamaica dogwood, lime flowers and wild lettuce. Any one of these or a combination of some of these will be useful although the stronger hypnotics are better for chronic cases.

Some of the commercial brands usually contain variations of some of these herbs although it is best to seek advice from a herbalist as more specific help will be given to identify the root cause of the insomnia and to fully address any underlying issues affecting the sleep pattern.

Other aspects of sleep are discussed in more detail in Chapter 5 (Health Essentials).

Irritable Bowel Syndrome (IBS)

One of the most common causes of lower abdominal pain in women which has posed one of the greatest challenges in clinical medicine with regard to definition and cause is Irritable Bowel Syndrome (IBS). It is often regarded as one of the functional bowel disorders. Symptoms range from periodic abdominal cramps, bloating, colic and bowel movements that alternate between constipation and diarrhoea. Frequently there may be mucous mixed with the stools. IBS is sometimes also referred to as spastic colon, spastic colitis, mucous colitis and irritable bowel. Most of these terms are misleading, for instance, colitis implies an inflammation of the colon which is not the case in IBS patients, leading to confusion with Ulcerative Colitis.

Surveys from the UK and the USA indicate that up to 20% of the adults in the Western World experience symptoms of IBS at some time. Most do not seek medical advice, but the chief unresolved question is whether those who do seek medical help have a different biological basis to those who do not, or is it an indication of a worried personality rather than disturbed gut function. It affects more women than men.

Since IBS encompasses a whole range of symptoms within inconsistent definitions of the condition, it is unlikely that it will be due to a single cause of organic origin but rather a combination of factors exacerbated in a susceptible individual.

Some of the factors implicated in IBS include the following:

- Foods (eg. Food Intolerance)
- Dietary Substances (especially synthetic eg. additives, preservatives, chocolates, milk products, alcohol etc…)
- Caffeine
- Inflammation & Infection
- Drugs & Medication
- Hormones (Menstrual Cycle)
- Seasonal Changes
- Stress
- Psychological Problems

Psychological stress and emotional responses to them can greatly influence GI function via the Brain-Gut connection. It is a well established holistic concept that true understanding of the Mind-Body link is the key to elucidating some of the more recent illnesses afflicting the Western World (such as the functional bowel diseases and chronic fatigue syndrome). The treatment of IBS is directed towards both the gut and the psyche. The diet requires review with those foods that aggravate symptoms being avoided. Current medical thinking about diet has changed a great deal in recent years.

An alternative therapeutic strategy for patients with significant pain is to use hypnotherapy or psychotherapy. Factors that favour a good response to psychotherapy include patients with predominant diarrhoea & pain, the association of IBS with overt psychiatric symptoms and intermittent pain made worse by stress. The relative advantages and disadvantages of cognitive behavioural therapy, interpersonal psychotherapy, relaxation/ stress management and pharmacotherapy are the subjects of on-going and controversial research.

The prescription of herbal remedies is supplemented with advice on dietary changes, patient reassurance and education. The holistic approach adopted by herbalists will enable the assessment of lifestyle choices and a psychological profile (ie. is there a predisposition to anxiety, depression or stress?) as well as the assessment of signs and symptoms in diagnosis and treatment.

Herbal remedies for IBS can range from the simple to the complicated; those with the following actions are indicated: antispasmodics for reducing the cramps in the gut, carminatives to getting rid of excess gas and bloating in the gut, demulcents to soothe irritated linings, astringents to reduce inflammation, nerviness to alleviate symptoms of anxiety and calm a worried personality. There are also a host of other herbs to improve the general digestive efficiency and anti-catarrhals to help clear mucus in the gut. Herb teas such as chamomile can be surprisingly effective due to its relaxation and gentle antispasmodic properties. Peppermint, ginger and fennel are all antispasmodics so they will relax the gut muscles that are causing the cramps. Herbalists often recommend combining herbs to make a single dose tea in order to soothe painful spasms and expel excess wind.

If the cause of IBS is much more deep-rooted than the mere symptoms, herb preparations are devised to address any psychological issues (eg. stress, anxiety, depression). Valerian is a popular choice due to its sedating and antispasmodic properties. Additionally, cramp bark can also be used to soothe spasms and relieve cramps. It also possesses a slight astringency which is believed to be effective against inflammation in the lining of the bowel. Goldenseal is primarily an antispasmodic but its other attribute is as a tonic to the mucous membrane so it will protect the bowel wall, helping to heal any areas of damage. It is particularly suitable for IBS management. A further benefit is that Goldenseal promotes the secretion of bile which aids digestion. Wild Yam is another useful herb with strong anti-inflammatory properties and is prescribed in IBS cases where a considerable number of painful spasms and passing mucus is a main feature of the condition. The prescription of very small doses of licorice is not uncommon since it is a powerful anti-inflammatory with laxative qualities. Moreover, herbalists believe that as with many other conditions, warmth can help alleviate the symptoms of IBS. Cinnamon is sometimes used to gently warm the bowel, while for a more robust effect, ginger is preferred. Both herbs also have a slight antiseptic quality that is helpful against inflammation. Another very useful herb is artichoke and this will aid digestion if food is proving difficult to digest. Other examples are listed below:

	Symptom		Useful herbs
(i)	Stress and Pain	(i)	Valerian or Chamomile
(ii)	Flatulence and Bloating	(ii)	Peppermint, Sage, Elecampane & Fennel
(iii)	Persistent Diarrhoea	(iii)	Add Raspberry leaves or Meadowsweet
(iv)	Persistent Constipation	(iv)	Add Dock
			(Add a demulcent : Comfrey, Marshmallow or Slippery Elm to all preparations)

J

Joint disorders

Joint disorders cover a wide variety of conditions such as arthritis (rheumatoid arthritis and osteoarthritis), gout, lumbago (backache) and osteoporosis. Lumbago, osteoporosis and gout are discussed separately. The main joint problem that people commonly experience is arthritis. There are essentially 2 types of arthritis, the type that is caused by 'wear and tear', through age and overuse of a particular joint called osteoarthritis and the type that has an autoimmune basis with complications affecting other organs and systems beyond the joint and this is called rheumatoid arthritis.

Both types of arthritis are characterised by joint swelling, pain, tenderness, heat in the joint and loss of mobility. The nodules that are often seen on the hands and other joints of the body is a classic hallmark of arthritis and this is usually the indicator of joint disorders but at this stage it is difficult to distinguish the type.

The herbal approach is to use a combination of herbs that tackle the pain and swelling whilst using internal mixtures to detoxify and cleanse the system in order to reduce the immune challenge that is resulting in inflammation. The long-term aim is to increase mobility and whilst there is no cure for arthritis, the focus is to manage the symptoms whilst improving the lives of many patients through pain management.

Herbs that are used topically include oil of wintergreen, cayenne pepper or prickly ash in a base cream of chamomile or arnica. Internally, supplements of devil's claw have had profound results as have turmeric and boswelia. Other herbs include white willow bark meadowsweet, prickly ash, nettle, Jamaica dogwood or devil's claw. As in all inflammatory conditions, it is important to look at the immune system since inflammation is very much an immune response, particularly in rheumatoid arthritis. Modulating the immune responses can be achieved through echinacea. However, liver herbs are equally important and in this respect, herbs such as dandelion and milk thistle are effective. Detoxification of any substances that are challenging the system can be addressed through burdock, cleavers or poke root, given in combination with good circulatory stimulants such as ginkgo to improve elimination. Bowel function is also important; a herbalist should be able to prescribe herbs that will optimise this function so as to prevent the build up of any waste or toxins in the system that could be the cause of inflammation.

Lifestyle changes such as gentle exercise (swimming and walking are both good for osteoarthritis and it is important to maintain joint mobility by taking exercise rather than letting them stay rigid). Some patients report that taking supplements of glucosamine sulphate and chondroitin sulphate helps as well as a sulphur based compound called MSM. It is best to seek the advice of a herbalist before buying any brand, especially products online which are not always regulated. Climate also helps and patients usually report that their condition significantly improves in the summer months. The key thing is learning to manage the condition and making attempts to be as mobile as possible and being able to do things without the constant agony of pain.

K

Kidney stones

Kidney stones are formed in a similar manner to gall stones. Salts or minerals form as crystals when the urine is filtered and in most cases, they are too tiny to be noticed. They pass harmlessly out of the body. However, in some cases, they can build up inside the kidney and form much larger stones and the problem happens when they pass from the kidney to the bladder along the narrow tubes and passageways. The pain can be sometimes excruciating. Complications happens when they get stuck, causing infection or rupture the linings or it can lead to permanent kidney damage. Other symptoms of kidney stones are sudden back ache, cloudy, bloody or smelly urine, feeling sick, an urge to urinate, fever and chills.

The herbal approach to treatment is really as a preventative measure since if the stone is known to exist, it will require urgent medical attention. Diet is closely examined since there are different types of kidney stones. In most cases, the cause is not known. However, insufficient water intake can concentrate the urine so increasing the risk of stone formation. Foods rich in calcium cause the most common type of kidney stones (calcium stones). Calcium stones are more common in people who have excess levels of vitamin D or who have an overactive parathyroid gland. People who have medical conditions such as cancer, some kidney diseases, or a disease called sarcoidosis are also more likely to develop calcium stones. Uric acid stones on the other hand are smooth, brown and soft. Excess amounts of uric acid can be caused by eating a lot of meat. Conditions such as gout and treatments such as chemotherapy can also increase the risk of getting uric acid stones. See under gout for more information on this condition.

Herbs commonly given for kidney stones are pelitory-of-the-wall, parsley piert and couchgrass. They combine well as teas with demulcent herbs such as cornsilk and marshmallow or urinary antiseptics such as buchu to prevent infection. In cases of previous kidney stones and to prevent further attack, it is best to consult a herbalist and a nutritionist to work out a long-term treatment strategy that incorporates dietary changes and herbal interventions. This may require liaison with the medical practitioner or doctor.

L

Laryngitis (see sore throat)

Leaky Gut Syndrome

Leaky gut syndrome is the term given to a condition where the gut wall becomes more permeable to food particles and other materials so much so that important nutrients are lost and cannot be absorbed effectively. The person becomes malnourished and illness sets in. Equally, toxins can also enter the system and cause an immune response – this leads to other problems particularly inflammatory conditions. Leaky gut is rarely acknowledged by doctors and so not routinely tested for. The condition may explain some of the many common symptoms people suffer from (eg. persistent headaches, bloating, poor digestion and abdominal pain) but are not attributed to this condition. It can also make an existing condition much worse, particularly inflammatory conditions such as arthritis.

The causes of leaky gut are many and varied such as insufficient stomach acid production, candidiasis, imbalance in the gut bacteria, stress, poor diet, alcohol and some medication.

The most effective long term strategy for treating this condition is through nutrition. Allergic and inflammatory responses to toxins or certain foods cause damage to the gut lining, resulting in holes that make it more leaky than normal. Therefore the first line of treatment is to identify these allergens and to avoid it. This will give the liver a chance to restore itself and to have a break from the constant role of detoxifying harmful substances that are being introduced into the system. Avoiding other culprit foods such as dairy, alcohol, processed foods, fizzy drinks and caffeine is also strongly advised. If there is an existing candida infection (thrush), it is best to avoid sugary foods including dried or canned fruit as this will only feed the infection and make it worse. Fermented foods containing yeast are to be avoided as is gluten (the protein from wheat). Foods that are recommended include the following:

- Organic vegetables and fruit (they do not contain artificial colours, preservatives or pesticides)
- Foods high in fibre
- Foods high in the essential fatty acids (fatty fish, walnuts, pumpkin seeds and flaxseeds)
- Drink plenty of water
- Slippery elm capsules will help restore the gut lining and heal some of the damage
- Peppermint tea has a soothing effect on the digestive system as does peppermint oil or capsules. Licorice and marshmallow can also be added.
- Prebiotic and probiotic supplements – they will restore the proper balance of the gut bacteria and protect the system against further damage
- Aloe vera juice – to heal any damage and a gentle laxative to clear out the bowels (this will eliminate the toxic challenge to the system and reduce inflammation)
- Chamomile tea to soothe and relax. Other relaxation techniques are also advised especially if stress is a feature of this condition.
- Infective causes need to be resolved by improving the immune system.
- A good multivitamin & mineral supplement in those that are substantially depleted of nutrients and are

evidently malnourished.

A consultation with a herbalist is strongly recommended.

Liver disorders

The liver is a powerful organ carrying out over 500 functions. The demands placed on it through poor diet and lifestyle means that the health of the liver is constantly compromised. Despite this, the liver possesses an extraordinary capacity to repair and regenerate so often that many of the consequences of poor diet and lifestyle take many years to develop and sometimes only manifest themselves in acute cases.

Many of us are more likely to be affected by poor liver function which can be easily resolved through diet, lifestyle changes and stress management. Liver sluggishness has a profound influence on health ranging from poor digestion, malabsorption of nutrients, poor sugar balance, energy dips and hormonal imbalance amongst other symptoms. At best, this can impair health and well-being, reduce vitality and mental alertness.

Liver disorders that are serious (eg. jaundice, liver cirrhoris, hepatitis) require specialist help in hospitals but it should be noted that in most cases, serious liver disorders can be prevented. A number of herbs are frequently prescribed by herbalists to repair and protect the liver. Good examples are dandelion and milk thistle which is usually included in preparation for most patients because liver function impairment is usually at the root of most common symptoms seen at clinic. Other examples include the Chinese herbs shizandra and bupleurum which work by neutralizing liver toxins. People who want a detox usually gain benefit from taking these herbs as well as others such as ginger, burdock, licorice and turmeric. Dietary changes are an absolute must. See earlier sections of this chapter for specific advice on liver function in health & well-being.

Lumbago (see backache)

This has been previously discussed under backache.

M

Macular degeneration

This has been previously discussed. See under eye disorders

Memory loss & poor concentration

This is a common problem and is usually symptomatic of age and decline. However, as we are now living longer than before (particularly in the West), degenerative disorders of the brain are becoming more common and occurring at a younger age than ever before. Memory loss and poor concentration can happen due a variety of reasons, biological disease being just one of them. Stress and illness can also affect the ability to think clearly, to remember important facts and details. At the more serious end of the spectrum, conditions like Alzheimer's disease (and a host of other dementia-related disorders) can be quite insidious in nature or rapid in progression leading to a profound impact on the lives of the sufferer and their families.

Mind exercises can help in the less serious cases as well as keeping up with activities and duties. Keeping the mind alert and active is extremely important so reading, knowledge-seeking and pursuing interests that occupy the mind and thinking will all help. Equally, reconciling oneself with past experiences, decisions and life experiences is also important as unfulfilled dreams, ambitions and unresolved issues can have a detrimental impact on a person's mental health and well-being.

The herbal approach to tackling this problem will be to examine all the details and causes. Treatment in a holistic context will involve the use of other therapies in conjunction with herbal medicine. Extreme and prolonged stress need to be tackled and a period of rest and recuperation after serious illness and debility. The herb ginkgo is very good at promoting circulation to the brain and the surrounding organs. A herbalist will also carry out a thorough review of diet and lifestyle and suggest changes that are practical and realistic in order to make the necessary improvements. A good, well-balanced diet is absolutely essential for brain function as is a balance between work and rest. Brain foods are a bit of a misnomer as all foods in the correct proportions have the potential to ensure good brain function. However, foods high in the essential fatty acids (omega 3, 6 and 9) are particularly important for healthy brain function. Suitable suggestions will be made specific to the person and lifestyle in question. There is no cure for degenerative disorders but with specific measures, it is possible to extend and improve the quality of life of loved ones so that their 'twilight years' can have some meaning and purpose.

Menopausal symptoms

Many women experience the discomfort of the menopause in the Western world. Typical symptoms include depression, hot flushes (also called hot flashes), weight gain, mood changes, anxiety, loss of libido, vaginal dryness (predisposing to cystitis) and insomnia to name a few. In theory, the menopause should be a relatively uneventful phase in a woman's reproductive life because the adrenal glands (which lie just above the kidneys) are the back-up glands for producing the all-important oestrogen when the ovaries start to slow down production of this hormone. Unfortunately, the stressful life that many women lead in the Western world leaves their adrenal glands in a depleted and exhausted state so much so that their back-up system fails and their bodies suffer the inevitable consequences of oestrogen decline and hormonal imbalance. Conventional treatments can range from drug therapy (eg. HRT) to radical surgery (total or partial hysterectomy). For some women, this appears to be acceptable and can alleviate much of their discomfort. However, many are uncomfortable with drug treatment or surgery and recent concerns over the safety of HRT have forced many to consider natural alternatives and less invasive methods of controlling their symptoms.

The herbal approach is to consider a range of herbs that tackle the problems on a more symptomatic level as well as a combination of practical suggestions or possibly even some of the talking therapies, particularly if the menopause occurs at an early age. Herbs that will control the hot flushes include sage and black cohosh. Herbs that control mood include St. John's Wort and other nervines such as skullcap, wood betony and damiana. Herbs for anxiety and insomnia include Indian ginseng, passion flower, lime flowers and Jamaica dogwood. Herbs that balance the reproductive hormones include false unicorn root, licorice, red clover or wild yam. A herbalist would prescribe the most suitable combination of herbs for each case so a consultation is strongly recommended. Diet is absolutely crucial so ensuring a well-balanced diet is critical to health at this stage. Getting the right balance of vitamins and minerals is important as well as slow-release, energy-rich complex carbohydrates. Much has been debated about soya and some of this information is confusing simply because some of it is contradictory and poorly referenced from non-reputable sources. Soya is one of the products that come under the general category of plant nutrients called phyto-oestrogens because when consumed, they exert an effect similar to the hormone oestrogen, although its action is weak. The table below gives further examples of other sources of plant oestrogens. In short, it is the fermented soya that is beneficial to health (whatever age but more so during the menopause). Fermented soya and their products such as miso, tempeh, tamari and shoyu are good examples. These reflect what is traditionally consumed in the Far East where menopause is a rare occurrence. Products such as soya milk, tofu (bean curd) and soya protein isolates are a Western invention and many argue that some of the health problems are attributed to the consumption of these products rather than the original soya preparation which are fermented. A consultation with either a clinical nutritionist or a medical herbalist is strongly recommended for comprehensive advice and guidance on this. Nutritional and lifestyle recommendation post-menopause is also advised such as preventing heart disease and osteoporosis.

Phytooestrogens

Over the last few years, there has been great interest in the role of naturally-occurring plant constituents that have a weak hormonal action in the body. These are collectively referred to as phyto-oestrogens (PO) of which there are 6 main types consumed by humans. POs occur widely throughout the plant world and can have a profound influence on human health particularly in oestrogen-deficient states such as the menopause. All types are naturally-occurring compounds and can be found in grains, seeds, legumes and medicinal plants in addition to other vegetable sources.

Classification of phyto-oestrogens; edible plants with recognised oestrogenically-active compounds:

PHYTO-OESTROGEN	COMMON SOURCES
Isoflavonoids • main ones = genistein & daidzein • glycitein in smaller quantities	• alfalfa • licorice[*] • mung beans • whole grains • red clover • soya[*]
Lignans	• linseed (flax)[*] • rye • legumes • beans • wholegrains
Saponins (similar structure to steroidal hormone oestrogen, progesterone & androgens. Some pharmaceutical companies use saponin-containing plants to manufacture steroid hormones)	• black cohosh – *Cimicifuga racemosa* • licorice[*] - *Glycyrrhiza glabra* • Korean ginseng – *Panax ginseng* • wild yam – *Dioscorea villosa*

• many medicinal herbs in this category • pharmacological mechanisms may involve interaction with hypothalamus-pituitary hormones rather than interaction with oestrogen receptors	• fenugreek – *Trigonella foenum-graecum* • root vegetables • grains
Coumestans	• alfalfa • soya sprouts* • green beans • kidney beans
Resorcylic Acid Lactones	• oats • barley • rye
Others	• fennel – *Foeniculum vulgare* • cabbage family • sage – *Salvia officinalis* • garlic – *Allium sativum*

Contains high levels of phyto-oestrogens

Menstrual cycle problems (irregular periods, missed periods, absent periods)

Menstrual irregularities are almost always a sign of hormone imbalance. In the absence of more serious pathology such as malignancy, this condition can arise from a number of things mainly poor diet, a stressful lifestyle and liver impairment. Menstrual irregularities creates a number of problems, particularly if fertility is an issue so regulating it is vital in a woman of reproductive age as well as to prevent and treat a number of distressing symptoms that accompany this condition. Hormone balancers are particularly indicated in these cases so herbs such as chaste berry, false unicorn root, Chinese angelica or black cohosh are useful. Improving the health of the liver is vital as this organ not only makes important hormones, it is also responsible for degrading them in order to maintain the fine balance of the various hormones. This has the effect of keeping the correct quantities of the relevant hormones in check so one or more do not exceed their limit, which in itself creates problems. Good liver herbs are dandelion, milk thistle, fumitory, goldenseal and burdock. Stress management and adequate exercise is vital as is a good diet. A consultation with a medical herbalist and a clinical nutritionist is needed to devise a diet plan and to address any nutritional deficiencies (which could also contribute to hormonal imbalances).

Mental health disorders

Mental health disorders can range from the mildest of anxiety or restlessness to more serious clinical depression, self-harm and dementia. Whilst herbalists can treat a variety of the less serious mental health disorders of the Western lifestyle, more serious problems require specialist help and/or counselling. There is no question that mental health problems of the Western world is on the increase, not assisted by a skewed value system and a strong emphasis on materialistic gain and a focus on individualism as opposed to the collective. A lack of spiritualism in this culture of Western decadent living has hampered many of the chance to be successful and happy. As a consequence, many are unable to reconcile themselves to this notion of living and their mental health suffers as a result. Depression is a classic example of this consequence and very much considered a 'Western' disease.

There are a range of herbs that can help in the symptomatic treatment but it is important to get a proper diagnosis and assessment from a specialist, GP, herbalist or other health care practitioner. Herbs that restore the nervous system include vervain, skullcap and wood betony. Herbs that help the system cope with stress include Siberian ginseng and Indian ginseng. Herbs that help in anxiety and tension include passion flower, lime flowers, valerian and chamomile. Herbs that have antidepressant properties include St. John' Wort and damiana. A healthy diet is vital to good mental health and well-being as is a proper balance between work and rest. Paying emphasis on spiritual health and well-being is critical to restoring harmony and a healthier perspective to life.

Migraines

Migraines are a specific and intense form of a headache which in some sufferers makes life unbearable because the pain is extreme. Why some people are prone to migraines is somewhat unclear although it does seem to run in families and women are more prone to attacks than men. In some people, making some simple changes and with herbal remedies can significantly reduce the frequency of attacks. The most important thing to identify is the type and character of the migraine as well as the cause or triggers such as food or lack of sleep. Once these have been established, the treatment is quite effective. The herb feverfew is a key herb given for this condition and many sufferers get much relief from taking this regularly. Other herbs of choice are wood betony, ginkgo, willow bark or cayenne. Butterbur has shown favourable results in recent trials. Triggers to avoid are certain foods (eg. chocolates, cheese, citrus fruits) caffeine (tea, coffee), alcohol, irregular or inadequate sleep, stress, irregular meals, smoking, loud noise, bright lights and extreme weather conditions. Women are more at risk because of the monthly hormonal changes. Balancing hormones with good diet and a healthy lifestyle is also essential.

Mouth & gum disorders

Symptoms of mouth and gum disorders can happen due to a number of reasons, dietary deficiency being one of them, particularly vitamin C. Taking adequate quantities of this (good sources are citrus fruits and potatoes) should get rid of symptoms such as bleeding gums quite quickly. However, other problems such as mouth ulcers, dental problems, bad breath and a furry tongue require specialist treatments as their causes are varied. Mouth ulcers in particular (aphthous ulcers) is quite a common problem. The most common cause is vitamin B_{12} deficiency but some people are more susceptible to this problem than others and it is not related to any nutritional deficiency. The herbal approach to treating this problem is to thoroughly review the diet and to identify any deficiencies in the diet. Herbs such as red clover, goldenseal, licorice and centella all help in healing the mucous membranes of the mouth. Other herbs such as sage, tormentil and witch hazel all help in astringing the membranes and so reduce the inflammation that accompanies mouth ulcers. Boosting the immune function is also important so a healthy diet is essential. Herbs that can help boost immunity include echinacea, ginseng and supplements of garlic. Ill-fitting dentures can also affect the mouth and gums so this needs to be examined in those cases.

Musculo-Skeletal disorders (sprains & strains)

Joint disorders such as arthritis have been previously mentioned. Muscular aches and pains, sprains and strains in the musculo-skeletal system are common especially in active individuals. It is also more common in the elderly through wear and tear of the joints with time and an increased susceptibility with age and decline. General weakness of the joints can be improved through specific exercises and a good diet. A consultation with a personal fitness trainer or a physiotherapist can be helpful in devising a simple exercise plan for strengthening the muscles around weak joints. Herbs that are useful in supporting the joints include nettle, juniper berries (topical application), St. John's Wort oil (topical application), cayenne pepper oil (topical application), horsetail and turmeric. Commercial muscle rub preparations containing arnica are most effective for muscular aches and pains, chills and strained muscles.

Supplementation that are recommended include glucosamine and chondroitin sulphate as a combination preparation, magnesium, a good antioxidant combination (Vitamins, A,C and E), calcium or vitamin D depending on the requirements.

N

Nausea & vomiting

Nausea and vomiting is not a common problem but it is a common symptom of so many conditions and side effects of medication. It is also common in the early stages of pregnancy. The treatment for this is very much dependent on the cause. In this respect, anything that remains when the obvious has been ruled out, especially if it is persistent requires a confirmed diagnosis from a doctor in order to determine if the problem is more serious and warrants urgent attention. Common herbs that are given for temporary nausea and vomiting are peppermint, black horehound and ginger. A combination of these in a tea form is frequently preferred by many patients.

Strategies to change eating habits, patterns, quantities and quality of the diet are advised. Any psychological or emotional issues also have to be addressed and this may require specialist help from counsellors or psychotherapists.

Nervous exhaustion

Modern lifestyles are increasingly hectic and many are subjected to enormous pressures in their attempt to balance home, work, family, friends and recreational or health pursuits. The classic term 'nervous breakdown' probably best fits the now modern term for nervous exhaustion or simply a 'burn out' (mental, physical, emotional and psychological). Many people continue for far too long coping with daily pressures and attempting to juggle a number of things or in some cases, leave issues unresolved and many questions unanswered because of the emotional pain of dealing with it in the first place. Stress, anxiety and worry can place a heavy burden on the weak and fragile individual and it is unsurprising that many face illness of the body and mind as a consequence of living in a globalised, fast and furious, modern 21st century world.

The herbal approach is to consider all aspects of the patient, their lives and the context in which they have fallen ill. Treating any symptoms can be effective in the short-term but a long-term strategy in some cases may involve talking therapies and additional support from other specialists and/or therapists. Herbs that support the nervous system include verbena, skullcap, wood betony or oats (to name a few). Any weakened system may benefit from the ginsengs, particularly in enabling the body to cope with stress and in encouraging the system to become more robust in handing everyday stresses. Reviewing the diet is essential and improving elimination, liver and digestive function also holds great benefit in a weakened state in order to prevent the build up of toxic material. Liver herbs such as dandelion and milk thistle may be useful as are digestive bitters such as bogbean, gentian or dandelion.

A general multivitamin and mineral supplement may be indicated in the immediate term as well as a vitamin B complex which is invariably depleted in weakened states. Devising a healthy diet plan is important in restoring the body's systems by getting the essential nutrients from food. Addressing lifestyle concerns such as incorporating an exercise regime into daily life, relaxation techniques, recreational pursuits and making time to 'switch off' is vital in restoring the body back to a healthy state. A consultation with a therapist, a herbalist and a nutritionist is highly recommended to work out a plan of action in tackling some of the long-term issues of 'burn out' and to prevent it happening again.

Nervousness (symptoms of) – see under anxiety

Neuralgia (trigeminal & post-herpetic)
Neuralgia is the medical term for nerve pain. The cause of nerve pain must be identified at the outset and this may require a referral from the doctor and diagnosis from the hospital to confirm any findings. Treatment will be much more effective if the cause is known but establishing this may be a problem in itself.

In a general sense, any organ or structure that is inflamed can press on surrounding structures and so trigger local nerves. This can produce the sensation of pain. However, two of the commonest types of nerve pain are trigeminal neuralgia (a type of 'stabbing' pain affecting a particular region on the face) and post-herpetic pain (a kind of pain that occurs after shingles, a viral infection that causes a rash across the chest and back region). This pain is more of a burning sensation. Herbalists are likely to treat both types of neuralgia. Herbs that are useful in alleviating pain include cayenne, St. John's Wort oil and arnica in topical preparations although treatment should be sought from a qualified medical herbalist. Internally, herbs such as vervain, Californian poppy or yellow jasmine are effective pain killers, lemon balm is good in protecting against viral infections as is St. John's Wort. Aspirin-like properties can be gained from white willow bark and meadowsweet. Many find herbal treatments useful in conjunction with other pain management therapies such as acupuncture and hypnotherapy. An additional herbal tea to calm and soothe the mind may also be helpful. A useful combination of chamomile, lemon balm, passion flower and valerian will also be sufficiently relaxing to encourage proper sleep as this may be disrupted as a result of intense pain. A consultation with a herbalist is highly recommended for specific advice and treatment preparation in each case.

Neurological disorders (eg. MS, motor neurone disease, restless leg syndrome)
Problems of the nervous system come in many forms. Some of them involve mental function, others involve aspects of physical ability and movement. Most of the common conditions are progressive (classified as degenerative disorders of the nervous system but this is not always the case). Two of the most common

neurological disorders that herbalists are consulted over are managing the symptoms of multiple sclerosis (MS) and treatments for restless leg syndrome. To cover all diseases of the nervous system is beyond the scope of the book so only these two will be addressed.

MS is a progressive, degenerative disease of the nerves producing variable symptoms from pins and needles to numbness and lack of movement. In some, symptoms can come and go and many go through periods of relapse and remission but in others the disease can progress quite quickly and patients deteriorate rapidly so it is an unpredictable condition. As this is essentially an inflammatory condition, herbal medicine aims to address this through reviewing fundamentals of elimination, digestion and immune function. Detox is not an uncommon strategy and some patients prolong their time in remission through clearing their systems of toxic build up which triggers inflammatory responses. Herbs that cleanse the system include senna or buckthorn bark although this needs to be supervised. Herbs that support the liver are dandelion and milk thistle. Immune herbs such as echinacea may be useful in modifying inflammatory responses and boosting the health of the immune system as in many cases, symptoms start after a viral infection. Other herbs that are generally nourishing for the nervous system include oats and rue. Increasing fibre in the diet is also needed as this will help elimination so flaxseeds and other sources from food are needed. There is some research to suggest that ginkgo can be useful in MS and supplements of vitamin B complex, B_{12} with folic acid, magnesium, vitamin E, vitamin C, copper and zinc. A consultation with a herbalist is recommended to devise a treatment plan for each case as this is such a variable disease. A healthy diet is essential in boosting general health and well-being and in making the system more robust and resilient.

Another common condition, is restless leg syndrome (RLS) which is a poorly understood condition producing spasmodic jerking movements of the leg, particularly at night and is often the cause of undiagnosed insomnia. Other symptoms include unpleasant sensations under the skin resembling a feeling of something creeping, crawling and/or tingling. It is sometimes painful and most common in middle-aged women, during pregnancy, those with severe kidney disease, iron-deficiency anaemia, diabetes, circulation problems, arthritis and nerve diseases. The herbal approach to dealing with restless leg is to address any underlying disorder such as those listed above as a first priority as symptoms will usually respond better from appropriate treatment. Excessive firing of the nerves can often be a sign of a restless mind so herbs that soothe, calm and nourish the nervous system can be useful. Examples include chamomile, valerian, lemon balm, passion flower and skullcap.

The general dietary advice is to reduce refined foods, especially refined sugar and refined flour, avoid processed foods with lots of additives, eliminate caffeine and restore normal iron levels; in short, attempting to restore the proper balance to the body. Other dietary recommendations include eating small, frequent meals, eating whole grains, nuts and seeds, fresh fruits and vegetables, and fish. In some people with RLS, the condition may be genetic (familial RLS) and responds well to supplementation of folic acid.

O

Obesity

Obesity is fast becoming a global epidemic despite the images we see of starving millions in certain parts of the world. The problem is more acute in the developed nations with other diseases associated with obesity such as diabetes and heart disease also on the increase. Certain cancers have also been linked to obesity and without doubt, the new crisis that is childhood obesity is going to present itself with a whole new set of medical consequences for the future.

To simply say that the treatment is to reduce food intake is not going to have any effective long-term benefits. Many have a psychological and emotional relationship with food and this needs to be addressed. This may require counselling or other talking therapies to resolve any underlying issues. A phased programme of gradual education and information is required so that the person can be re-programmed to eat healthier foods and incorporate an exercise regime. By far, the most effective, safest and long term solution to being overweight is diet and exercise in combination. Fad and fancy diets may have short term benefits in weight loss in those that are marginally overweight but for the clinically obese, therapies involving counselling or psychotherapy is required alongside advice and support from a nutritionist and a herbalist. Family counselling may also be necessary.

Osteoarthritis (OA) – see under joint disorders

Osteoporosis

This is a disease of the bone often referred to as brittle bone disease. The bone mineral density is significantly reduced causing the bone to become fragile and brittle. They have an increased risk of fracture and breakage so people affected by it need to take extra care. Typically, fractures can occur in the back, hip and wrist. It is particularly common in post menopausal women and the elderly but it can also be caused by various other hormonal conditions, smoking and steroid medications and many chronic diseases.

Conventional treatment involves supplementation of vitamin D and calcium and in some cases, hormone replacement therapy is considered. The herbal approach would be to ensure adequate intakes of calcium and vitamin D through natural food sources such as dairy, especially milk. However, this needs to be in moderation along with other good sources such as dark green leafy vegetables, avocado, fatty fish, liver and nuts. Exposure to sunlight is necessary as the body relies on this to make vitamin D. Also, thirty minutes of weight-bearing exercise such as walking or jogging, three times a week, has been shown to increase bone mineral density, and reduce the risk of falls by strengthening the major muscle groups in the legs and back. It is important to be shown how to do exercises for osteoporosis by a professional physiotherapist; this will ensure that the sufferer gains full benefits and does not cause further damage.

Ovarian cysts – see under Endometriosis and PCOS (polycystic ovarian syndrome)

P

Pancreatitis

Pancreatitis is inflammation of the pancreas, an important gland that produces a range of digestive enzymes and hormones that control blood sugar levels. Symptoms can come and go depending on how severe the inflammation is and whether the condition is chronic where the pancreas becomes permanently inflamed. Symptoms include severe abdominal pain especially when lying down, nausea, vomiting and fever. Gallstones and alcohol cause the majority of the cases of pancreatitis but there are other less common causes such as viral infections (eg. mumps). In cases of severe pain, hospital treatment is a must. Herbs that reduce inflammation such as chamomile or licorice are good choices as are herbs that heal and soothe irritated membranes such as mullein and goldenseal. Supplementation of vitamin C and selenium is highly recommended especially in chronic cases but essentially, it is better managed within conventional medicine so the condition can be closely monitored and pain can be more effectively managed as strong doses of conventional analgesics may be required.

Panic attacks – see under anxiety

PCOS (polycystic ovarian syndrome)

Polycystic ovarian syndrome is a problem of the ovaries and essentially due to a hormonal imbalance. It is characterised by a number of cysts in the ovaries and accompanied by irregular and light periods, weight gain, acne, excessive hair growth and infertility. Many sufferers have a greater or lesser extent of these symptoms so the condition is referred to as a syndrome, a collection of symptoms. In cases of excessive weight and insulin resistance, weight loss can help because sugar balance is restored and the demand for insulin reduces. Diabetes and being overweight as well as a family history are all risk factors in this condition.

The herbal approach to this problem is quite complex and requires a thorough review of the symptoms, the context and history of the condition is needed. Herbal hormone balancers such as chaste berry are necessary to regulate the menstrual cycle and to counterbalance the excess oestrogen in this condition. Other hormone herbs include black cohosh, false unicorn root and wild yam. They mimic the body's own oestrogen and produce weak effects by blocking the receptor sites for the body's more powerful and stronger hormone. Balancing the hormones has other desirable effects such as reducing hair growth, regulating the menstrual cycle and eventually to encourage the production and release of mature eggs. This will address problems of fertility which is a common symptom of PCOS. Good choices are white peony, licorice and chaste berry. There are other herbs which different patients respond to so a consultation with a medical herbalist is strongly advised so that an effective treatment plan can be devised in each case. This will address all the symptoms that are a feature of this condition such as insulin resistance, weight gain, diabetes and the stress-related symptoms that often accompany this condition.

Peptic ulcers

Peptic ulcers are very similar in character to duodenal ulcers except that they happen in a different location in the gut, tending to affect the upper part of the stomach, near the entrance rather than the latter part, near or in the duodenum. The symptoms include pain in the top part of the abdomen, nausea, vomiting indigestion and belching. On a long-term basis, there is weight loss (because eating becomes associated with symptoms so many sufferers begin to limit food) and iron-deficiency anaemia due to blood loss when the ulcers penetrate the gut wall and rupture local blood vessels and surrounding tissues. However, this is not that common because symptoms would be severe or the condition would have to be chronic, recurring over a long time. Severe pain would require emergency hospital treatment.

The causes have been linked to poor diet, stress and a poor lifestyle. There is an association with a bacterium called *Helicobacter pylori* and certain medications like anti-inflammatories (especially drugs like aspirin and other non-steroid pain killers). One of the causes is the lack of production of the mucus which protects the stomach lining from the eroding effects of the stomach acid. The herbal approach to treatment is to firstly encourage the lining to heal and restore balance to the stomach environment. This requires some supplementation of probiotics (particularly those containing *Lactobacillus* species) which contain important numbers of the healthy bacteria which will outnumber the *Helicobacter pylori* species. Healing the gut lining will require herbs that soothe and reduce the inflammation. Herbs with demulcent and anti-inflammatory action such as licorice, marigold and marshmallow are all good choices. These are best taken as a tea. Goldenseal (either as tablets or tea) is great at healing a damaged gut wall and slippery elm powder will soothe and calm irritated linings, it is particularly effective at reducing the burning pain that accompanies this condition.

Dietary changes such as cutting out alcohol, spicy foods and fried foods is advised as is not eating late at night, limiting fibre and stopping smoking. Stress management is advocated where it is a strong element in the case. Supplementations of turmeric, vitamins B complex, vitamin C and zinc can be useful but it is best to seek help from a medical herbalist before self-medicating.

Period pain

Some women suffer excruciating period pain whilst other women have very little pain, and at best a mild discomfort. Period pain is caused by muscle cramping that limits blood flow to the local area. General exercise can help reduce the monthly pain because it promotes the production of the body's natural painkillers (a group of chemicals called endorphins). However, specific exercises designed to improve the blood flow to the pelvic region may help further. Herbal antispasmodics and painkillers such as cramp bark, Jamaica dogwood pulsatilla, valerian and yellow jasmine are effective in some women. Tonics to the uterus are also helpful and these include raspberry leaf and black cohosh amongst others. Increasing blood flow to the pelvic area can be useful too so herbs such as yarrow, ginkgo or ginger would be helpful. Diet is essential as eating a wholefood diet free from additives and preservatives and plenty of fresh fruit and vegetables will provide all the right nutrients to maintain a strong body. Supplementations of vitamin B-complex, B_6, calcium and magnesium may also be needed.

Lifestyle measures would include specific exercises, particularly the aerobic type and stress reduction measures such as relaxation techniques, massage therapy and meditation.

PID (Pelvic Inflammatory Disease)

PID is quite literally an inflammatory disease of the pelvic region, that is, inflammation of the ovaries, uterus and fallopian tubes and the surrounding tissues. The cause is infective, usually bacterial infection such as chlamydia and gonorrhoea. Infection can be through sexual contact, childbirth or a gynaecological procedure such as a termination. PID must always be treated immediately as the consequences and complications of untreated symptoms can lead to infertility, toxic damage to the surrounding tissues and organs and the increased risk of ectopic pregnancy.Symptoms include an unusual discharge, irritation of the vulval lining, lower abdominal pain and sometimes fever. In some cases, there are no symptoms. Recurring PID is either a consequence of poor education, information and poor sexual practices or poor immune function and personal hygiene.

Herbal treatments include echinacea, garlic, thuja, horsetail, dandelion and yarrow. Blood cleansers will remove toxins in the system that provokes an inflammatory response so herbs such as violet, parsley and red clover are good. For irritation in the local area, herbal tea mix that includes marshmallow or cornsilk will be soothing. It is important to look at elimination too as build up of waste (toxins) will continue to trigger the inflammation. Other measures require radical changes to sexual practices, education, stress reduction techniques/relaxation methods and cutting out smoking as this increases the risk. A consultation with a medical herbalist is highly recommended for proper advice and an effective herbal treatment plan.

Pins & needles

Many of us have suffered pins and needles. In the most simple cases it is caused by pressure or compression of the nerve that supplies the local area of the body resulting in a tingling sensation and numbness in the affected parts. It is also caused by previous nerve damage (injury or surgery), disease or trapped nerve. These will require special attention in managing the symptom and in identify the underlying cause. Pins and needles can also be a symptom of iron-deficiency anaemia which requires a thorough investigation into the cause and supplementation with iron in the first instance. Herbs that are good for the nervous system include skullcap, chamomile, devil's claw and ginseng. Supplementation of vitamin B_6 will also help.

PMS (premenstrual syndrome)

PMS covers a wide range of symptoms from bloating and irritability to pimples, sugar cravings and breast tenderness. Some of the known symptoms are listed below:

- Fatigue and tiredness,
- Listlessness or lethargy
- Headaches or migraine
- Depression and low mood
- Sleep disturbances
- Nausea, bloating & other digestive complaints
- Emotional, feeling vulnerable, low concentration and other mental health symptoms
- Mood changes
- Sugar cravings
- Breast tenderness and/or pain

- Skin symptoms such as acne, poor pallor or a dull complexion

Not every woman experiences the symptoms of PMS and it is widely acknowledged that it is not a normal physiological process. For those that suffer the symptoms, not all of them experience the same set of symptoms hence it is referred to as a syndrome (a collection of symptoms attributed to this phenomenon). Herbalists usually classify the symptoms into a particular profile in order to make treatment more effective and to address the long-term issues involved in each case.

PMS is essentially a consequence of a hormonal imbalance. Many factors affect the regulation, production and timing of hormonal secretion that is associated with the menstrual cycle such as stress, diet, environment and emotional events. In the first instance, it is very important to establish whether the symptoms have a cyclical nature since the diagnosis of important conditions (such as clinical depression for example) can be easily missed under the umbrella of PMS.

Herbs can be given to treat the symptoms but usually, regulating the menstrual cycle and improving liver function is a good start. Hormone balancers such as chaste berry have shown excellent results. Herbs that promote oestrogen are sometimes recommended too such as licorice, sarsaparilla and false unicorn root. Liver herbs such as dandelion and milk thistle are recommended to prevent toxic congestion such as headache and ear blockage. The adrenal glands also need support and herbs such as licorice and borage are useful. Many have reported the benefits of evening primrose oil but a reputable brand is essential. Herbal diuretics such as celery, boldo leaf or nettle will address some of the bloating that occurs due to water retention. Other symptoms can be addressed specifically such as antidepressants to lift mood (eg. St. John's Wort), address some of the stress and fatigue with the ginsengs and sleep disturbances with nervine relaxants and sedatives (eg. passion flower, valerian or lemon balm). Supplements are also advised such as the essential fatty acids (flaxseed oil, hemp seed oil), magnesium vitamin B_6 and vitamin E. Dietary modifications should include limiting alcohol, dairy foods, refined carbohydrates and sugars, processed foods, limit or avoid stimulants especially caffeine and increase complex carbohydrates, fibre and vegetables. More about these and examples of these types of foods are given in Chapter 5 – Health Essentials. A consultation with a herbalist is strongly advised to determine the type of PMS and the best treatment plan for each case.

PMT (premenstrual tension)
This forms part of the symptoms of Premenstrual Syndrome (PMS), please see above.

Poor appetite
Poor appetite can be a sign of something more serious so it should always be regarded seriously. However, children are sometimes very fussy eaters and usually complain of a lack of appetite. It is best to leave them until they are hungry as they will make it clear when they want food! The elderly are another group who typically have a poor appetite. This is because their digestive function diminishes with age and the digestive juices and sense of smell that trigger a good appetite is reduced. Herbs that are useful include herbs that have

a particularly bitter taste. Examples include bogbean, wormwood, gentian and dandelion. Stress, diet and lifestyle should also be looked into and making changes such as regular exercise, reducing stress, limiting alcohol intake and stopping smoking could all benefit. A consultation with a medical herbalist would help as they will make helpful suggestions for change and identify key problem areas and cause(s) of the problem. A prolonged bout of poor appetite or even a loss of appetite requires further investigation through the GP or consultant specialists following investigations.

Prostate problems/enlargement (BPH)

BPH stands for benign prostatic hyperplasia and is the most common problem of the prostate gland, particularly in middle-aged men. It is potentially a concern because it could lead to cancer so it needs to be regularly monitored. Symptoms are urinary infrequency and hesitancy, and should be distinguished from prostatitis which is an inflammation of the prostate gland caused usually by a bacterial infection. The exact cause of why this happens is not yet certain.

By far the most popular herb for BPH is saw palmetto which works in the same way as the commonly prescribed conventional drug (finestride, traded as Proscar®) and has been widely used in Europe since the 1930s. The herb has great appeal in the Europe as well as America being one of the biggest selling herbs on the market. Extracts of saw palmetto berry are being used extensively throughout the world for the relief of BPH. Supplements of selenium and zinc are highly recommended as are other herbs such as buchu and bearberry which generally support the urinary tract system. Cranberry juice or supplements of it may also be advisable. It is best to consult a herbalist on reputable brands to get the best benefits of the herbs.

Psoriasis

Psoriasis is a fairly common dry skin condition characterised by flaky, thickened patches of skin that are covered in silvery scales. They are most frequently found on the elbows, knees, lower back and the scalp but it can occur almost anywhere on the body. In some cases, the condition can be intensely itchy and can produce a burning sensation. The cause is unknown and the condition is often aggravated by stress and complicated by arthritis.

There are a number of treatment approaches that a herbalist would use depending on the case, the severity, the type and symptom profile. The stress element is also reviewed as in many cases, it has been shown that onset has been triggered by a stressful event about 4 weeks prior. In essence, the herbal approach is to improve digestion, particularly protein digestion (so bitter herbs such as gentian, dandelion or wormwood may be given) and then to work on clearing the toxins from the system (so herbs such as burdock, blue flag or yellow dock can be chosen). Importantly, it is good to support the circulatory system in removing these toxins to the excretory organs so a herb such as ginkgo would be a good choice. The most notable herbs for this condition however are mahonia (Oregon grape) and sarsparilla although it is still not fully known how they work in clearing up the symptoms in psoriasis. Other herbs could include licorice and calendula as they are both soothing to the skin..

Dietary measures must address food sensitivities and examine and review all aspects of diet and lifestyle. Increasing essential fatty acid (vegetable sources of omega 3 and 6 oils) intake is advised as is avoiding all acid-forming foods especially those that are high in protein such as meat, eggs and fish. Recommendations include increasing the intake of vegetables and fruits and to limit or avoid tomatoes, potatoes, aubergines and cayenne pepper. Also, to take a probiotic supplement, live yoghurt and increase water intake. A consultation with a medical herbalist is strongly recommended in the first instance, and a clinical nutritionist if a specific and detailed diet programme is indicated.

R

Raynaud's syndrome or disease
This is also known as Raynaud's phenomenon characterised by an intolerance to the cold producing an adverse reaction in the extremities of the body such as the fingers and toes. Blood vessels in these regions of the body constrict excessively leaving the fingers and toes numb, cold, blue and swollen. It is a disorder of the immune system affecting more women than men. The condition is more common in migraine sufferers and often, treating the migraine can significantly reduce the symptoms. Herbs that improve the circulation to the surface of the skin such as ginkgo, cayenne and ginger help a great deal. Others such as rutin and prickly ash are also helpful as are supplementations of calcium, evening primrose oil and vitamin E. Dietary measures include avoiding red meats, dairy, stimulants (tea, coffee) and cold drinks with ice. Practical measures such as wrapping up well in cold weather, wearing protective gloves or heated gloves and having regular hot meals.

Renal colic
Renal colic is a type of pain caused by kidney stones. Causes of kidney stones have been discussed (see above). Renal colic pain is colicky in nature affecting the kidney area and radiating through the sides to the bladder. Pain management for small stones is required until it is passed out but for larger stones conventional treatment or intervention is required.

Repetitive Strain Injury (RSI) – see carpal tunnel syndrome

Respiratory disorders (asthma, hayfever, bronchitis, pneumonia)
Some people are more susceptible to respiratory conditions than others. Addressing the underlying causes is vital since establishing the allergic or infective component to each condition will have an influence on the focus for the treatment. Asthma, bronchitis and hayfever have all been discussed (see above). Pneumonia is a serious condition that warrants conventional medical attention in the first instance. It is an inflammation of the lungs caused by an infective agent and antibiotic treatment will clear the infection. Herbal treatment is usually to restore balance to the body particularly in the body's defence to infection and in boosting respiratory health. Lingering symptoms can include cough, muscle weakness, debility and muscle pain in the chest area. Herbs such as elecampane, coltsfoot, hyssop, hawthorn, elderflowers and yarrow are all good choices. Muscle rubs containing cayenne pepper oil, comfrey, eucalyptus oil and rosemary oil ease breathing and soothe the aching muscles in the chest region. Boosting the immune system with Echinacea and wild indigo should be given together with supplementations of garlic, vitamin C and zinc. A good probiotic may also be advised to get digestive function back to normal. A consultation with a medical herbalist is strongly recommended.

Rheumatism & rheumatic conditions

Rheumatic conditions cover a wide range of symptoms and are often associated with the elderly although this is not always the case. Generally, it encompasses inflammatory disorders of the muscles, joint stiffness and various forms of arthritis. Some of these have been previously discussed (see joint disorders, gout and backache). Treatment will very much depend on the condition but general supplementation with fish oils, glucosamine sulphate, chondroitin sulphate and significant dietary and lifestyle changes, particularly if a strong association between them has been established. A consultation with a herbalist is recommended in the first instance for a diagnosis of the condition before treatment, advice or supplementation is given.

Rheumatoid arthritis (RA) – see under joint disorders

S

Sciatica

This is a painful condition caused by a trapped nerve (the sciatic nerve) that radiates from the lower back to the back of the legs down to the calf region. Injury, wear and tear, poor posture and arthritis could all be possible causes of sciatica.

Inappropriate firing of the sciatic nerve happens when the vertebrae through which the sciatic nerve runs collapse on each other and cause pressure on the nerve root. A common cause is a slipped disc and patients are usually advised bed rest once the pain and numbness has gone. Treatment is based on the cause and attempting to remove it by making changes if possible eg. changes in posture, limiting repetitive movements, taking care with back injuries especially in previous episodes of a slipped disc etc... Topical rubs and massage oils can help and preparations include herbs that have an anti-inflammatory, analgesic and heating effect. Good choices are cayenne pepper, arnica, clary sage oil, prickly ash, St. John's Wort oil and wintergreen. Tincture mixtures can be prepared to be taken internally and could include herbs such as devil's claw (good anti-inflammatory and analgesic), white willow bark (anti-inflammatory and analgesic), yellow jasmine (analgesic but has to be under the supervision of a herbalist), ginkgo (brings blood to the affected parts for increasing healing) and other measures such as acupuncture, massage therapy, deep tissue massage or chiropractic.

Sexual dysfunction (also see Erectile Dysfunction)

Sexual dysfunction is a complex issue and one that cannot be tackled fully here. In men, it can take many forms but predominantly it results in impotence, or more commonly referred to as erectile dysfunction (ED). Natural products, particularly herbal remedies have a long tradition of use worldwide for this problem and has resulted in many studies being carried out into how effective they really are for patients. Loss of libido and ED need to be thoroughly investigated for cause as this could range from diet, stress, injury, illness, drugs (including alcohol), medication, emotional or psychological issues.

Sexual dysfunction in women is more to do with loss of libido which is the general term applied to the instinctive drive associated with sexual desire. This can vary from one individual to another and particularly in women, this can be to do with many factors from psychological and emotional to the physical (eg, loss of libido after pregnancy or during the menopause). Loss of libido requires specific help and possibly counselling if no physical cause can be identified.

Herbs such as Korean ginseng, damiana, centella, sarsaparilla, ginkgo and saw palmetto can all be useful. Lesser known herbs such as the muira puama plant, *Tribulus terrestris* and yohimbe bark have been used traditionally in some parts of the world and are now being commercially marketed. It is best to seek the advice of a qualified herbalist before self-medicating on any of these commercial preparations which may not have been regulated or tested for their benefits or safety.

Treatment could also benefit greatly from other therapies such as the talking therapies, couples counselling or psychotherapy depending on the cause of the problem. Diet and lifestyle will have to reviewed thoroughly too. Poor diet, lack of exercise, too much alcohol, stress and tension in a relationship can all profoundly affect sexual function. To determine these, a consultation is required which may involve referral to a specialist.

Sinusitis

Sinuses are air-filled cavities lined with mucous membranes that are found in the skull bones. Sinusitis is an inflammation of these membranes which is almost always caused by an infection. This produces pain, usually in the forehead region, on either side of the nose and on the cheekbones. Fever and general upset can also happen. The cause of the infection must be addressed, particularly if this is a recurring problem. In some allergic states, the mucous membranes can become inflamed and cause similar symptoms. Sinusitis is usually a problem of congestion and poor immune function. Infection occurs in susceptible cases and clearing the congestion to ease breathing and to get rid of the pain is the main focus.

Herbs such as eucalyptus oil, menthol, myrrh and camphor are great at dilating the air passages so ease the breathing and congestion. These are best taken by steam inhalation. A herbalist may also be able to prepare a rub or lotion containing any of the above herbs as well as eyebright which can be applied to the sides of the nose, underneath the nostrils (to ease breathing) or on the forehead.

Chronic cases of sinusitis require a radical look at factors that promote the symptoms. Immune function needs to be improved as do digestive and liver function to improve elimination of waste material and reduce congestion.

Other measures involve getting a good diet that is balanced and healthy (to include garlic, ginger and cayenne as spices into daily cooking – they are great natural antibiotics), exercising regularly, avoiding a smoky environment, avoiding stress and taking appropriate measures to manage it, taking the appropriate medication if there is an allergy (eg. hayfever). A consultation with a herbalist is strongly recommended in chronic or recurring cases as the choice of herbs will depend on the symptoms and the severity of the condition.

Skin disorders

Various skin disorders have been discussed under their specific headings. Some require specific treatments to address the root causes such as regulating immune responses responsible for an inflammatory condition, increasing essential fatty acid intake in dry skin conditions etc… However for good skin health a good diet, a good circulation to the skin and a healthy digestive system is vital (as are other aspects).

Further aspects of good skin health are discussed in Chapter 5 (Health Essentials).

Sleep disorders

The importance of sleep has been discussed in previous chapters (see Chapter 1). The most common sleep disorder is insomnia which covers a range of symptoms from a disturbed sleep to not being able to fall asleep. Insomnia has been described above.

Sore throat

A sore throat is caused by a bacterial infection and it may be recurrent in those who have a weakened immune system and are generally run down. It may also be part of a wider set of symptoms such as the common cold and usually signals an infection in the upper respiratory tract or the surrounding associated structures such as the ear or nose.

For immediate relief, a gargle made from diluted tinctures of sage, oak, witch hazel, myrrh and tormentil may help. Teas or other preparations using herbs such as thyme, licorice, elderflower and echinacea may help with any respiratory tract infections (see treatment for common cold). Supplements of vitamin C and zinc may be necessary to boost the immune system in cases where this is recurring and to examine the diet and lifestyle thoroughly to restore balance and banish the main stress factors in the case.

Stress (symptoms of)

Each person copes with stress in different ways. Some experience great stress without any visible sign or symptom of ill health whilst others suffer immediately with things like frequent colds, insomnia, skin outbreaks or rashes, an exacerbation of stress-related disorders such as eczema, migraine, IBS etc… There are so many conditions that are profoundly affected by stress and so many symptoms can be attributed to it. Once the link between stress and a particular symptom has been established, then effective measures can be made to combat the stress.

The ginsengs, particularly the Indian ginseng (also known as ashwagandha) and the Siberian ginseng are especially useful in stress as they enable the body to cope better and modify the body's responses to stress. The adrenal glands need extra support during stressful times so herbs such as licorice or borage may be useful. In most cases, it is advisable to adopt stress reduction or stress busting measures and exercise is one the best ways to do this as it encourages the release of endorphins (the body's natural relaxant and mood enhancer). Meditation, yoga, tai-chi and other recreational activities may be useful too. Learning to cope with stress is also vital as no doubt modern life is extremely stressful and there is no getting away from it. Making our mind and body more robust at handling this is the first step in preventing the recurring symptoms of stress.

T

TATT (Tired All The Time)

Being tired all the time can signal a number of things. It is important to rule out more serious conditions such as malignancy, anaemia or metabolic disease to name a few. Being tired all the time however, as opposed to exhausted (which most serious illnesses cause) is usually a sign of system failure, being run down and a general decline in body function. On a simple level, examining the diet and lifestyle, stress factors and immune function can reveal a lot. A radical overhaul is required on all levels if there its persistent tiredness.

In the first instance, dealing with the tiredness, taking Korean ginseng or Siberian ginseng can help boost energy. Rosemary has a stimulating effect and nerve tonics such as skullcap or vervain are very useful. Nutrient herbs such as oats or alfalfa are good at restoring balance in depleted systems. A multivitamin and mineral supplement may also be required to restore depleted stores of essential nutrients in the initial stages of treatment. Of course, this will have little long-term effect if it is not properly supported by dietary measures such as ensuring a healthy, balanced diet that is fresh (wholefoods, preferably organic) and an avoidance of processed foods or foods loaded with additives. Stimulants such as tea and coffee should also be avoided as this will further deplete the adrenal glands and affect the production of energy. Stress is another cause of tiredness so it must be addressed (see above). Supporting the liver is also important because it will help the body derive the best nutrition from the foods eaten so herbs such as dandelion, milk thistle and burdock will be useful. A consultation with a medical herbalist is highly recommended in order to establish the cause of the tiredness and then to work out a phased programme of treatment that considers each case specifically according to the patient profile.

Tension headaches – see under migraine and headache

Thyroid disorders

Thyroid disorders are complex and their diagnosis is ever more complex compounded by the fact that it does not always reveal the true extent of the problem. Nevertheless, thyroid disorders are usually classified as either under active or overactive. Hyperthyroidism and Hypothyroidism have been discussed earlier in this section. The thyroid gland makes an important hormone (thyroxine) which regulates the rate at which we mobilise energy from the food we eat. In other words, it controls our metabolism. A chemical signal from the brain activates the production of this hormone so any disorder of the thyroid gland can also be due to problems in the brain signal. The herbal approach to addressing thyroid abnormalities is to establish whether the problem is at the point of the gland or at the brain. It may be that in some cases, a referral may be necessary if tests are required. Some of the symptoms may also be addressed directly in conjunction with treatment for the thyroid disorder.

An under active thyroid can be diet-related due to an insufficient intake of the mineral iodine, which is a component of the thyroid hormone. It may also be triggered by hormonal fluctuations especially in women. This may happen at times when the body is under the greatest hormonal changes such as adolescence, pregnancy or menopause. Symptoms include weight gain, extreme lethary, exhaustion, fatigue and tiredness, the need to sleep, depression, poor body temperature regulation, hair loss, poor immune function, IBS, arthritis, dry skin, constipation and a goitre (a swelling in the neck due to an enlargement of the thyroid gland). Kelp (also known as bladderwrack) supplements are great at increasing the metabolic rate and is often prescribed for an under active thyroid. Increasing the intake of iodine-rich foods is also necessary if it is due to a dietary deficiency. Iodine can be found in seafood and sea salt. Some foods like bread, milk and cheese have been fortified with iodine so it is best to check the label. Other nutrients are also important.

These include the essential fatty acids, zinc, vitamins A, C and E as well as a vitamin B complex. General tonic herbs that are stimulating such as the ginsengs and rosemary may also prove useful in boosting energy levels.

An overactive thyroid can be caused by autoimmunity (antibodies being made against it) and so increasing the production of the thyroid hormone. It could also be caused by an overabundance of iodine in the diet, food allergies, a leaky gut, stress or infections of the bowels. Symptoms include weight loss, palpitations, excessive sweating, anxiety and muscle tremors. Other symptoms may include, diarrhoea, brittle fingernails, itchy skin, insomnia and a goitre. The herb bugleweed (also known as gypsywort) is usually the herb of choice in suppressing an overactive thyroid gland. Another useful herb is horseradish. A good diet and establishing the cause is vital as is getting a healthy balanced diet with the right proportions of the essential nutrients.

A consultation with a herbalist is required in the first instance to assess the symptoms and to make or confirm a diagnosis associated with the thyroid gland. Some liaison with the doctor may also be required in some cases.

Tinnitus – see under ear disorders

Tonsillitis
The tonsils are part of the immune system and are made up of glands that respond to infection. Tonsillitis is an inflammation of these glands and they are situated at the back of the throat. Both bacteria and viruses can cause an infection and the tonsils respond to this infection by the swelling that is observed. This response gives other characteristic symptoms of tonsillitis such as sore throat, fever, pain on swallowing, headache, discharge from the tonsils and general malaise.
The conventional treatment for bacterial tonsillitis is a course of antibiotics although this is not effective against viral infections. Recurrent tonsillitis is usually a cue to have them removed. This may lead to a susceptibility to throat infections or mouth ulcers later on as the tonsils are a secondary immune organ and do protect the local environment against infection. The herbal approach in the first instance is to boost immunity by giving herbs such as echinacea, ginseng or astragalus. A gargle made of diluted tinctures of sage, witch hazel, tormentil, myrrh or oak to reduce the inflammation then a mixture of demulcent herbs at a later stage when the pain of inflammation has reduced to soothe and restore the mucous membranes. Good choices of herbs could include slippery elm, licorice, mullein or marshmallow.
Boosting immunity and making it more robust is a priority in recurrent infections therefore ensuring a good diet is essential. A supplement of Vitamin C and zinc is also advised.

Toothache
Toothache can be caused by a number of things and it is important to establish whether the problem lies in the teeth itself or at the gums. Problems of the gums have been previously discussed (see under mouth and gum disorders) and in some cases, may require conventional treatment. Problems of the teeth really require

specialist dental care and treatment. Toothache can be caused by dental cavities and only a dentist will be able to treat that. In bacterial infections that cause pain, one of the best home remedies is to rub a few drops of clove oil onto the tooth and gum area. This will numb the area and so alleviate the pain. Also, a freshly cut garlic clove can be rubbed onto the affected area. Toothache can happen due to poor dental hygiene and possibly combined with a reduced immune system that does not fight off infection easily. Immune boosters such as echinacea and goldenseal as supplements may be needed to prevent further attack and infection. In all cases, it is best to have a check up with a dentist who will be able to make an early detection of the more serious problems which only they can treat.

U

Ulcerative Colitis (see under Inflammatory Bowel Disease)

Ulcers

Ulcers can appear at common sites in the body through various causes. The common ones that occur in the mouth are called aphthous ulcers and this has been previously discussed. Those that appear in the gut lining, especially in the stomach (peptic ulcers) and duodenal (duodenal ulcers) regions have also been discussed (please see under the relevant heading). Then there are those ulcers that appear on the skin often as a complication of a wound or an infection that is slow to heal. A herbalist would be able to prepare ointments of St.John's Wort oil, comfrey, chickweed, slippery elm goldenseal, aloe vera or marshmallow. Honey is also a good choice both internally and externally. Teas containing echinacea, dandelion and burdock can be useful as well as supplementations of garlic, vitamin C and zinc.

Under active thyroid – see under thyroid disorders

UTIs (urinary tract infections) including urethritis

The urinary tract consists of the kidneys, the ureters, the bladder and the urethra. Urinary tract disorders will involve any one of these structures, the common ones being infections (UTIs). Regardless of the therapeutic approach, it is imperative to initially address the symptoms (without which complications could arise) but also to view the underlying mechanisms and risk factors to prevent recurrence at any level. Symptoms can include pain in the lower abdomen, lower back, hip region or upper thighs, a burning sensation when passing urine or blood in the urine which will require immediate attention.

A common UTI in women is cystitis and in men it is urethritis. Herbal treatments aim to address the symptomatic relief of pain and discomfort whilst tackling bacterial numbers. In this respect, a variety of urinary antiseptics prove valuable in providing safer alternatives to the current antibiotics. Good choices include nettle, bearberry, goldenrod, cornsilk, couchgrass and horsetail. Some of the herbs are soothing to the irritated linings so will reduce some of the discomfort when passing water. A supplement of cranberry extract is also highly recommended.

V

Vaginal dryness

Vaginal dryness is usually a symptom of the menopause. Lubrication that is normally secreted when young starts to decline as the production of the hormone oestrogen starts to decline. This happens during the menopause but the worst effects of it can be limited or even prevented with a good diet and maintaining a lifestyle that combats stress.

Since oestrogen is in decline, herbs that mimic the actions of the hormone are indicated. This includes wild yam, licorice, red clover and black cohosh. Additionally, dietary intake of fermented soya (miso, tempeh, tamari) will limit the symptoms of menopause. Essential fatty acids are vital to ensure the skin and mucous membranes are healthy and adequately protected. This can be taken as supplements such as hemp seed oil or flax seed oil (as part of oil dressings for salads) or as tablets/capsules. Topical skin preparations may also help by directly moisturising the area and so preventing the membranes from drying out. Herbal preparations may contain centella (oil), marigold, chamomile or licorice (creams) with hemp seed oil added in accordingly for a soothing and moisturising cream. Herbs may be prescribed to address the other symptoms of the menopause. For cases of vaginal dryness that is not associated with the menopause the hormone profile of the patient must be reviewed in order to determine the underlying causes of hormonal imbalance. This may require further tests and diagnosis.

Varicose veins & varicose ulcers

Varicose veins are swollen veins that occur most frequently on the calves of the legs due to loss of the valve function in the blood vessels. This means that there is a backflow of blood that accumulates in the vessels, causing a swelling which can sometimes lead to infection and ulceration. They are more common in older women although anyone is at risk who has a weak blood vessel health. This includes those who are overweight, pregnant, a family history of weak valves in the veins. Other factors such as age and standing long hours in the day all contribute to this condition. The herbal approach to treating this condition is to thoroughly examine all risk factors, diet and lifestyle. Support stockings and raising the legs while at rest are practical measures that are useful and some cases may require surgery.

Herbs such as horse chestnut, butcher's broom, hawthorn, witch hazel and horsetail are all good choices although it is best to see a herbalist for preparation as sometimes a topical cream may need to be prepared. An extract of pine bark called pygnogenol has shown extremely good results in recent trials for varicose veins and in poor blood vessel health. Herbs and supplements that are high in bioflavonoids (good antioxidant activity) will boost the health of the blood vessels. Bilberry, ginkgo, red berry, grapeseed, pine bark are all good choices. A herbalist will be able to devise an effective treatment plan that includes herbal supplements as well as practical measures such as regular exercise and keeping mobile.

Varrucas

Verrucas are warts that occur on the soles of the feet. They are the same as warts on any other part of the body. However, they may look different because they may have a more flattened appearance. Verrucas are caused by a viral infection through skin to skin contact so it is more common in gyms and swimming baths. Good personal hygiene is essential to limit the spread of infection.

Herbs that are effective at reducing the size of the wart are thuja (tree of life), greater celandine and marigold. Tea tree and other antiviral agents such as echinacea, garlic or goldenseal will all help to eradicate the wart. With the exception of tea tree (which can only be applied topically), all the others can be taken internally or externally. A consultation with a medical herbalist is highly recommended.

Vitiligo

Vitiligo is a skin condition caused by the loss of pigmentation due to the destruction of the cells that produce them. It is believed to be an autoimmune disorder where the body attacks its own tissues. Gradual de-pigmentation of the skin can start on the face, hands and feet, and progress to other parts of the body and become more widespread. The herbal approach to treatment is to clear the body of toxins and waste as this triggers the immune system. Herbs such as poke root, cleavers, burdock or yellow dock will all do the trick of clearing the system. A good circulatory system herb such as ginger or ginkgo is needed to assist the removal of these toxins to the organs of waste. Equally, good liver herbs such as dandelion and milk thistle are also required.

Boosting the immune system is also needed as this may have become depleted or maladjusted due to overload. Herbs such as echinacea or marigold may be useful here. Topical creams of aloe vera gel or comfrey cream are well tolerated over time and are safer for long-term use. They are preferred by patients over the standard steroid creams that are prescribed by doctors since steroid creams can thin the skin and cause skin damage. Dietary supplements of vitamin C , B complex and the amino acid phenylalanine is also needed.

As this condition can be quite disfiguring, it is important to address the emotional side of things as the symptom can be very distressing to patients. Herbs such as valerian, lemon balm, chamomile and passion flower may all help soothe and relax. A consultation with a medical herbalist is highly recommended.

W

Warts

This has been discussed under verrucas. The same treatment approach applies to all warts.

Water retention

Water retention (fluid retention) in the body has a number of causes and produces a number of problems. In essence, it is the body's inability to remove excess fluid from cells and to eliminate them from the body. As a consequence the body retains more fluid (mainly water) than it needs and can result in weight gain, swollen fingers, ankles and high blood pressure amongst other things. The latter is more serious but it can be easily remedied if it is to do with excess water in the body rather than other causes. More serious causes of fluid retention is associated with heart failure which will require treatment and assessment from conventional doctors. The most common cause of water retention is too much salt in the diet. To maintain the balance in the cells and tissues, the body retains water so that the excess salt does not cause disruption to the chemical balance that is needed for body processes to work. However, water retention can also be caused by hormonal imbalances (eg. PMS), poor sugar balance, poor liver function, food intolerances, excess toxins in the body and lack of exercise. Diets that are very low in calories (especially proteins and other important nutrients) can also cause water retention.

Herbal diuretics such as dandelion leaf, boldo and celery and can all be very effective at removing the excess water in the first instance but this should be under supervision because overuse of diuretics can deplete important nutrients and further disrupt the balance. Prescription of herbal diuretics is usually accompanied by proper advice about diet and lifestyle. A consultation with a medical herbalist is strongly recommended in order to assess the underlying factors such as heart function, blood pressure and nutritional status.

Weakness and debility

This describes the subjective feeling that patients experience in many chronic, long-term and severe conditions where the body is substantially depleted of energy and nutrients leaving the patient in a weak and vulnerable state. Root causes are infection, strenuous work or undue demands on the body, mental stress and acute or chronic disease including the common cold. Debilitated states require a comprehensive and co-ordinated treatment plan that takes into account the immune status, the cause of the debility, nutritional status and physiological function. In the immediate term, herbs that boost energy levels and are a general tonic may prove useful. These could include herbs such as Korean ginseng, rosemary, damiana or sarsaparilla. Oats is a great herb for general weakness and debility as it strengthens and nourishes the nervous system and contains a range of important nutrients. In the long term, addressing immune function which may have become weakened and impaired, is crucial to improving defence and in ensuring a more robust system. Herbs such as astragalus, echinacea or Siberian ginseng will be useful here. Nutritional status is vital in restoring balance and repairing damaged cells and tissues, replenishing systems so that they can function better. Levels of hydration also need to be examined as well as the electrolyte balance as this will determine how cells are functioning and any impact on blood pressure. The impact of stress on the person is also important as prolonged and sustained stress can deplete the body of important reserves and eventually, the body just runs on empty until it cuts out. Combating stress is a major part of modern living and some do it very successfully, others not so well. A consultation with a medical herbalist is highly recommended so that an effective treatment plan can be devised which takes into account all factors that have led to this point of weakness and debility. A diet plan and lifestyle changes will be advised as well as herbal tonics and energy boosters that will address the immediate problem whilst providing suitable, practical measures to prevent a recurrence of things that have led to this state in the first place. This may require a radical change in thinking and behaviour.

Weight disorders (overweight, weight loss, underweight)

Almost everyone has experienced weight fluctuations and in Western societies where there is such an unhealthy obsession with weight and appearance, it is becoming ever more common for people to experience weight disorders. Interestingly, there are two ends of the spectrum here; whilst obesity is fast becoming a global epidemic, there is also a strand of individuals who are clinically underweight or anorexic. Then there are those who have 'issues' with food and adopt unhealthy eating habits such as binge eating, abuse of laxatives or regurgitate their food etc... by means of having some control in their lives or in an attempt to deal with emotional issues. For most of these individuals, there is almost always a psychological relationship with food which may represent various things to them. Extremes in weight (either clinically obese or anorexic) requires psychological intervention and support along with re-education about food and professional help from a herbalist, nutritionist or a dietician to change habits, possibly from a lifetime. An examination of the environment, stress levels and genetics is also required as each may have an influence on the regulatory processes that maintain a healthy weight.

It is important to note that in weight loss regimes, the tried and tested method of a healthy diet combined with adequate exercise is the only effective long-term solution to weight loss. There are no quick fixes and no shortcuts to long-term weight loss. No herb as yet has been proven to be the miracle weight loss herb but with professional advice from a herbalist, herbs can be extremely useful in assisting the body in losing weight. In this respect, it is important to examine factors such as water retention, sugar balance, metabolic rate, hormone balance, quality of the diet and exercise patterns (type, duration and frequency).

Sudden weight loss that is not intentional should always be investigated and an appointment with the GP is advised in the first instance. Sudden weight gain can be a number of things (such as side effects to medicines or pregnancy for example) but if this is unintended, again it needs to be investigated. People with weight disorders need to consult a medical herbalist who will be able to devise an individual treatment plan that includes diet and lifestyle changes that are realistic and manageable.

Wounds

Wounds can be internal or external. Internal injury requires treatment at hospital after consultation and treatment from doctors. External wounds can be severe in which case, it requires hospital treatment. However, minor injury to the skin and superficial wounds respond extremely well to herbal treatments. Herbs that are wound healers include marigold, comfrey, aloe vera, centella and marshmallow amongst others. Nutritional supplements such as vitamin C and E as well as zinc are recommended for wound healing. Internal mixtures of centella and horsetail along with circulatory stimulants such as ginkgo and bilberry will be very useful.

X

Xantholasma

This is the fatty deposits of cholesterol that are formed around the eyelids and joints (tendons) in people with high cholesterol levels in their blood. See under hypercholesterolaemia for treatment. Also known as xanthelasmata.

Y

Yeast infections

Yeast infections display similar symptoms to the most common yeast infection candidiasis (thrush). See under this for treatment.

Z

Zinc deficiency

Zinc is a mineral that is essential for healthy function of the body. It helps with the healing of wounds and is part of many chemical reactions in the body that are assisted by enzymes. It is vital for the healthy working of many of the body's systems and is particularly important for healthy skin, wound healing and restoring skin integrity in inflammatory conditions such as eczema and psoriasis. It is absolutely vital for proper functioning of the immune system and in ensuring effective resistance to infection.

Symptoms of zinc deficiency include recurring infections (a sign of poor immune function), skin problems (eczema, psoriasis, acne and others) and a reduced sense of taste. Other symptoms can include hair loss, diarrhoea, fatigue and poor wound healing. It is always best to get all nutrients from food and zinc is present in a wide variety of foods, particularly in association with protein foods. A vegetarian diet often contains less zinc than a meat based diet and so it is important for vegetarians to eat plenty of foods that are rich in this vital mineral. Good sources for vegetarians include dairy products, beans and lentils, yeast, nuts, seeds and wholegrain cereals. Pumpkin seeds provide one of the most concentrated vegetarian food sources of zinc. In patients who are significantly zinc deficient and have symptoms of zinc deficiency, medicinal doses of 15mg a day is required but this has to be monitored by a health practitioner and not through self-medication. For normal healthy adults, the recommended intake is 9.5mg for men and 7mg for women.

(iii) Women's health and herbal medicine

Women are more inclined to seek help (alternative or conventional) when it comes to their health. It is unsurprising therefore that herbalists are consulted more frequently by women than by men for a range of conditions. It is also undoubtedly true that women have more to contend with regarding health and well being simply because of the complexity of the female system, the hormonal profile, the reproductive system and all that that dictates in addition to the many pressures that face the modern female patient.

There are a range of herbs that are commonly used for 'female problems' notably in generating a better mood and easing the symptoms of stress including reproductive problems and sexual health. These are predominantly the areas most treated but it's not to say that there aren't many others. In addressing these common female problems, some herbs are used time and time again, with effectiveness. More often than not, the conditions that I frequently treat in women have an emotional element that warrants specific help. In this respect I keep a regular stock of the following:

- St. John's Wort – great antidepressant and anxiolytic
- Dandelion – great liver herb, diuretic and digestive herb
- Siberian ginseng – great at helping the body cope with stress
- Chaste berry – good for regulating hormones and combating the symptoms of PMS
- Black cohosh – great herb for menopausal symptoms (commonly seen at clinic)
- Sage – great herb for hot flushes

- Echinacea – excellent all round immune booster (best as a prophylactic)
- Skullcap – great nervine; soothing and calming frayed nerves
- Ginkgo – great circulatory booster and good for brain function
- Lemon balm – great for stress, anxiety and viral infections
- Passion flower – great for stress and anxiety
- Lime flowers – reduces high blood pressure, relaxes and calms. Good for anxiety

I always advocate some form of exercise to all my female patients. I think this is particularly important in this climate as there are many demands that face women and expectations of women are very high in our society. Stress levels are also abnormally high and this can lead to all sorts of complications regarding the hormonal balance which is one of the first things to go out of sync (so to speak), and particularly during stress. Exercise will not only offset the worst excesses of stress and anxiety but also improve a woman's self-confidence and esteem by improving aspects of her physical health and mental well-being. It will also encourage more positive feelings about body image, appearance and physical fitness.

Many of my female patients struggle to find a good balance in their lives, be it due to work pressure, family commitments or personal time. Many of them seek alternative ways of living (and working) to seek this balance, and much of this about personal growth and development in as much as practical solutions to common dilemmas. Many find exercises such as yoga very useful in addition to other measures such as biofeedback, spiritual healing and meditation. Others find help from a life coach/ a NLP practitioner or a counsellor helpful. Much of the work of a herbalist is about giving guidance, advice and healing beyond the physical ailment and encouraging women to celebrate life and themselves in addition to finding practical help to common ailments affecting them.

(iv) Men's health and herbal medicine

There are a host of herbs that can help with the many ailments that affect men. The health of many men is compromised far more frequently because of neglect, a poor diet and an unhealthy lifestyle rather than any other factor or genetic predisposition. Therefore many of the problems affecting men can be easily remedied through making simple changes. A herbalist can certainly advise in this regard.

There are few things that specifically affect men but in general, improving immunity (to protect against infection) is key as is their mental well being. Many men harbour problems for a long time and are notorious at keeping quiet about it, refusing to seek help until it becomes a medical emergency. However, the trend is slowly changing and many men are keen to maintain a certain level of health and well-being, adopting practices and measures to optimise their health.

Of the many conditions that I see, there are common symptoms that men tend to seek help far more than others. These include poor immune function, recurrent infection, boosting or restoring energy levels (requiring a general herbal tonic or stimulant) and BPH (see above). Currently, there is an increase in the incidence of testicular cancers and men are encouraged to have this checked on a regular basis. Occasionally there are allergic conditions, autoimmune disease and chronic inflammatory conditions but these are not as frequent as the others.

Men need to take particular care over their digestive function and mental well-being, both of which become significantly compromised with age and decline. Acknowledging the problem is the first step towards recovery and this may require the help and intervention of family, friends and other loved ones. Given the current crisis in the major economies of the world, recession and expectations of men in providing for their family, there are a number of common themes of which the greatest is the compromising of their mental health & well-being. Depression, suicidal thoughts or a desire to self-harm and an overwhelming feeling of inadequacy are becoming increasing common.

(v) Children's Health and herbal medicine

The formative years for a child are the most critical. All aspects of learning, behaviour and psychology are all important in a child's development and a well-informed parent is as crucial as the access to treatments, advice, information and availability. This also applies to health and well-being. Good nutrition, a happy and healthy environment for a child is as critically important as the other aspects of child development.

Children suffer more than most from recurrent infections, primarily because their systems are not fully developed and this includes their immune system and their liver. A healthy diet, free from additives and preservatives, clean air, a peaceful environment and plenty of exercise is absolutely vital to children's physical health and emotional well-being. The good thing about children's health is their capacity to make a quick recovery which is immense because their systems are relatively unpolluted through prolonged exposure to toxins and bad habits. It is also where I have seen that herbal medicine works at its best and most effective. Common ailments that affect children have been discussed in more detail under the specific problems above and under herbal first aid.

(vi) Health as you get older

The health of the elderly warrants a special mention as there are many things that can be done to enhance and prolong health and well-being, well into old age. Many of the problems that are symptomatic of age and decline can be avoided through a healthy diet, a healthy lifestyle and through supplementation. Many physiological functions start to deteriorate and some of the things taken for granted in youth (like having energy for instance) is simply not there anymore. A pragmatic approach to life and accepting one's physical limitations is a good starting point and this will avoid disappointment and a certain frustration that accompanies a state of mind that tries to do more than the body will permit.

Keeping the mind active, keeping physically active (within one's own limitations) and cultivating different skills, hobbies and pastimes will all help in improving the quality of life as we get older. Western societies place an unnatural and unhealthy emphasis of youth and does not value age and experience. As a consequence, many people worry about old age and start to feel devalued and useless. This is not only unnecessary but also a cruel injustice to a group in our society who have so much to offer by way of wisdom, skills, knowledge and the all important life experience.

CHAPTER 5 – HEALTH ESSENTIALS

(i)   Mood, sleep and energy (inner well-being and fitness)
(ii)   Skin, hair, nails and feet
(iii)   Spine and posture
(iv)   Important aspects of nutrition

(i) Mood, sleep and energy

Mood, sleep and energy and all interdependent, that is, they all depend on each other to be at optimum level. When your sleep is disrupted or insufficient, then mood and energy levels are low, a person can become irritable and concentration is limited. When energy levels are low, then mood and sleep are both affected. When mood is low, then sleep is affected which in turn has a profound effect on energy levels, particularly if the situation is sustained or prolonged in any way.

To combat the worst excesses of these problems, it is important to maintain all three at an optimum. There are a number of ways of achieving this and there are many practical measures that can be taken to ensure that this state of being is maintained.

First of all, identifying the causes of stress, anxiety, disruption to sleep, altered mood and changes in energy levels can all help. There are those instances however, that some of life's stresses are unavoidable and so, our responses to them must be reviewed and changed if mood, sleep and energy are to remain at an optimum. Each of these aspects needs to be examined in its own right as each has a profound impact on inner health and well-being.

Mood and Mental Well-being

A positive approach to life can be extremely difficult, particularly when problems appear to engulf us or situations become overwhelming or intolerable. Many have sought the help of life coaches and NLP (neuro-linguistic programming) practitioners, some have found talking therapies helpful and others seek solace from simply talking to someone close. Establishing a network of help is important as it would avoid the need to feel isolated and thinking that there is no-one to go to for help or advice.

Mercifully, cultural changes in our society have dictated that we talk more readily about our problems than generations before us. It has become socially more acceptable for us to display emotion and to discuss quite openly about matters of the heart or other issues that perhaps our parents and grandparents simply accepted and just 'got on with it'. This does not make the current generation feeble or weak in any way; on the contrary. Current demands and modern life in the 21st Century mean that it is not easy to remain positive, optimistic and hopeful in the face of huge pressures, financial commitments, worry about debt, an aggressive marketing culture and an increasingly materialistic world with skewed value systems that makes us all feel inadequate and unfulfilled. It is hard to resist any of these pressures but with a sturdy support network and a strong spiritual basis, it is easy to maintain a positive outlook on life and avoid the daily stresses that often grind people down.

In more recent times, mental health and wellbeing has warranted much attention, particularly now in recession-hit times and the realisation of modern governments that unbridled capitalism does not work. Whilst wealthier nations of the world (such as the US and the UK) have long enjoyed material wealth for some time, they remain spiritually poor and in desperate need of a sea-change in attitude, thinking and behaviour. Despite the few and rare exceptions, we have lost our capacity to think as a collective, as a society and consideration of fellow human beings for the benefit of humanity as a whole. The selfishness and mindset of many for some considerable time has impacted on those who do not fit into or adhere to this way of thinking with the inevitable consequences on their mental health.

Depression is fast becoming a big social issue. In the UK, a leading mental health charity estimates that the current statistic for depression is 1 in 4 soon to be 1 in 3. Other mental health problems such as anxiety are also on the increase. To avoid the symptoms and long-term consequences of such disorders, there have to be strategies to combat the problems before it is too late and serious illness sets in. With regard to depression, many people find that doing charity work has an enormous benefit to their mood as the concept of helping others in a less fortunate situation than themselves provides them with great consolation and a sense of purpose which they could not identify with before. It can speed up the process of healing a great deal by the mere act of giving and helping.

Life coaching is becoming increasingly popular as is NLP as a means of effecting change and setting important goals for success (whatever area of life that may be). NLP can be considered as a collection of information and techniques that enable changes or improvements in thinking, behaving and feeling. This may have many benefits from improving self-esteem, confidence, having the ability to communicate effectively and acquiring the necessary skills to make significant changes.

The concept of happiness is also important as is developing one's spiritual health which is often neglected in the buzz of daily living and modern lifestyles. Inner well-being and fitness is absolutely dependent on self-esteem, confidence, a sense of contentment or happiness and being at peace with oneself. Many aspire to achieve this state for many years and are constantly 'searching' for spiritual strength and peace. The route to achieving this is not difficult or out of reach for anyone. A change in perspective, engaging with people and a proper value system that does not place an unhealthy emphasis on material gain is the essential starting point.

Sleep

The importance of sleep cannot be adequately emphasised. The nature of sleep and its purpose has been briefly described in Chapter 1. Current statistics put women at the top with regards to sleep disruption with 1 in 3 being affected by disrupted sleep or not being able to fall asleep. Regular lack of sleep has a profound impact on health and the long-term consequences can lead to depression, irritability, headaches, impaired reflexes, reduced mental alertness and physical tiredness amongst other symptoms.

Sleep can be affected by a number of factors such as:

- Anxiety & worry
- Pain (various causes)
- Illness (various)
- Hot flushes & other menopausal symptoms
- Hormonal fluctuations (may affect production of melatonin, an important component in determining the circadian rhythm/body clock of the body)
- Mental illness eg. depression, anxiety, post-traumatic stress disorder
- Stress
- Other factors & outside influences eg. noisy neighbours, uncomfortable bed, partner who snores
- Medication
- Diet (quality of food and timing of meals)

Additionally, variable shift work has a negative effect on the body. A variable shift pattern does not allow the body to adapt sufficiently and this interferes with the natural body clock (the circadian rhythm). Consequently, hormones are disrupted and the body is in a constant state of change. It's a bit like being in a perpetual state of jet lag which, on any long-term basis, is not beneficial at all to the body.

The solutions to tackling disrupted sleep depends very much on the nature of the problem, establishing a cause and effect and deep-rooted issues which may require specialist help such as counselling for depression, specific help for emotional trauma etc… Some of the strategies could involve the following:

- Examining diet and lifestyle
- Adopting a holistic approach to the problem. Examine all aspects of:
    - Mind (mental well-being)
    - Body (physical well-being)
    - Spiritual well-being
    - Psychological well-being
- Other measures to relax & unwind
- Effective pain management
- Meditation, tai chi & other stress-busting measures
- Other intervention eg: counselling, massage, hypnotherapy, reflexology etc…

Diet is an integral part of ensuring we get a good night's sleep. Some of the foods to avoid and some foods that need to be increased are highlighted below:

Foods to avoid	Increase intake of these foods
Biscuits, cakes, chocolates & others foods that are high in refined sugars	Green vegetables except spinach
Coffee, tea, cola drinks, chocolate drinks & fizzy drinks (too much caffeine)	Lettuce (natural sedative)
Red meats, rich creamy dishes & cheese (high in protein & difficult to digest especially late at night)	Porridge (slow-release carbohydrate will regulate sugar and energy levels)
Spicy dishes, curry or oriental foods (can cause heartburn which will disturb sleep)	sunflower and pumpkin seeds (high in magnesium – will relax muscles, relieve stress and promote sleep)
Alcohol & tobacco (disrupts body processes and generally bad for health)	Wholegrain foods & other low glycaemic index (GI) foods (eg. wholewheat foods, brown rice, oats). These regulate blood sugar levels, calm & soothe the gut & nervous system.
Bacon, ham, sausages, sauerkraut, spinach & tomatoes (all increase adrenaline which will keep the body alert at night so that it is difficult to get to sleep)	Increase complex carbohydrates in wholefoods (eg. pasta) boosts serotonin levels which in turn promotes sleep. Serotonin is regarded as the body's natural relaxant & antidepressant.
	Cottage cheese, turkey, yoghurt, bananas & avocado (foods high in tryptophan which is the precursor to serotonin. This in turn promotes sleep.

Lifestyle changes also need to be made in cases of stress, lack of exercise and other issues such as emotional trauma, depression, anxiety and worry. Examples of appropriate measures include:

- Stress management – stress has a huge impact on the quantity and quality of sleep. Stress busting measures will not only address the physical effects of stress but also ensures mental and psychological well-being, which in turn will enable proper sleep. Good examples of stress management techniques are yoga, meditation, aerobic exercise, recreational pursuits, hobbies or simply socialising with friends. All are great ways to combat stress. This will restore efficient functioning of body processes such as hormone regulation which, if disrupted, has a profound and negative impact on sleep.

- Exercise – regular, aerobic exercise is a great way to combat the negative effects of stress, depression or anxiety, all of which affect sleep. In addition to the physical and mental benefits of exercise, sleep will be more regulated as the body can become tired at regular times due to exercise and this will encourages a proper sleep pattern. A calm and relaxed body and mind will positively promote sleep.

- Herbal help – many have sought relief from a range of herbal supplements, teas, herbal remedies and OTC preparations specifically designed to calm, soothe, relax and sedate the mind and body. Notable herbs include chamomile tea, hops, valerian, passion flower, lemon balm, Californian poppy, lettuce and St. John's Wort amongst others. These are considered to be herbal sedatives and hypnotics, all of which promote sleep. Their advantage over prescription drugs is that they promote better attributes of sleep without the unwanted side effects such as feelings of grogginess the morning after. Before self-medicating however, it is strongly advisable that the true cause of sleep disturbances is correctly identified so that important issues such as depression, anxiety or emotional trauma does not go undiagnosed and effective treatment is sought. This will eventually have the effect of indirectly resolving any sleep disorders which may well be a symptom of these underlying problems.

Energy

Energy is critical to health and well-being. There are a number of things that can affect energy levels. Nutrition is one of the main factors and this is discussed later. Mental well-being is also vital as this can deplete important energy reserves so it is useful to examine 'energy-wasters' such as depression, anxiety and stress, and ways of combating these problems. Equally, energy boosters can be enormously helpful and apart from the nutritional element to boosting energy levels, there are other measures such as exercise, mood, spiritual health and acquiring peace of mind. Rest and relaxation is also important and must be balanced with sufficient work challenges and mental activity that staves off boredom (another source of energy depletion). Appropriate breathing, particularly deep breathing will also boost energy. So exercises that promote efficient oxygen exchange at the lung surface through specific breathing techniques will assist in getting the all-important oxygen to cells and tissues. This will promote better energy production.

Herbal energy boosters such as rosemary, the ginsengs, damiana, St.John's Wort and echinacea can be very helpful in some cases plus supplements of vitamin B complex or indeed an all round multi-vitamin and mineral in cases of malnutrition. It is best to seek proper advice first from a medical herbalist or a nutritionist before self-medicating as each case needs to be reviewed in its entirety so problems that are affecting energy can be correctly identified and addressed. Foods that deplete energy are having too much caffeine (tea, coffee, fizzy drinks), not enough water, low calorie foods, too much fast foods and refined sugars, alcohol, chocolate and in some cases, too much wheat.

Stress and nervous exhaustion have a significant impact on energy levels and as such, nutritional support is strongly advised. Good nutrition is also essential to recovery. Further details on specific foods that are advised for optimum health are highlighted later. This also holds true for nutritional help in post-viral fatigue and nervous exhaustion. Other general and important considerations include the following:

- Examining the fluid and electrolyte balance eg. levels of hydration, salt & sugar balance
- Examining the quality and quantity of the nutrient intake

- Macronutrients (carbohydrates, proteins, fats)
- Micronutrients (vitamins, minerals & others eg. co-enzyme Q_{10}, probiotics, bioflavonoids, phyto-oestrogens)
- Examining fibre intake (body is not designed to store waste and any build up of toxins due to low fibre intake will affect the body negatively and make unnecessary demands on the body)

Fatty acids intake:

There has been a lot of media coverage on the subject of the essential fatty acids and how good they are for you. We are apparently not getting enough of these nutrients from our diet due to the appalling standards of the 'western diet' having too much of the unhealthy saturated fats, hydrogenated fats and refined sugars. To understand the true importance of essential fatty acids, it is perhaps best to start at a description and their function in the body.

The essential fatty acids (EFAs) are a vital part of our diet because they cannot be made by the body, so they need to be obtained from the diet. In this sense, they are therefore referred to as 'essential'. They are a group of fats (lipids) and make up some of the most important parts of our body especially the brain, hence the term 'brain food'. There are 2 types of essential fatty acids that are important – omega 3 and omega 6. There is also omega 9 but this is not technically essential as the body is capable of making it provided there are enough of the other EFAs in the first place. The EFAs are needed by the body in certain proportions; more is needed of the omega 3 than the 6. Omega 3 is found in flaxseed oil (flaxseed oil has the highest omega 3 content of any food), flaxseeds, flaxseed meal, hempseed oil, hempseeds, walnuts, pumpkin seeds, Brazil nuts, sesame seeds, avocados, some dark leafy green vegetables (kale, spinach, purslane, mustard greens, collards, etc.), canola oil (cold-pressed and unrefined), soybean oil, wheat germ oil, salmon, mackerel, sardines, anchovies, albacore tuna, and others.

Omega 6 is also found in flaxseed oil, flaxseeds, flaxseed meal, hempseed oil and hempseeds. Other sources include grapeseed oil, pumpkin seeds, pine nuts, pistachio nuts, sunflower seeds (raw), olive oil, olives, borage oil, evening primrose oil, black currant seed oil, chestnut oil, chicken, amongst many others. It is important to avoid refined and hydrogenated versions of these foods. Other sources must be checked for quality as they may be nutrient-deficient as sold in stores. These include corn, safflower, sunflower, soybean, and cottonseed oils which are also sources of omega 6, but are refined and may be nutrient-deficient.

Omega 9 is found in olive oil (extra virgin or virgin), olives, avocados, almonds, peanuts, sesame oil, pecans, pistachio nuts, cashews, hazelnuts, macadamia nuts, etc. One to two tablespoons of extra virgin or virgin olive oil per day should provide sufficient omega 9 for adults. However, the "time-released" effects of obtaining these nutrients from nuts and other whole foods is thought to be more beneficial than consuming the entire daily amount via a single oil dose.

For a clear mind, a healthy body and efficient use of energy, the essential fatty acids are a vital part of the diet. They also have other health benefits such as maintaining the suppleness of the joints, offering some protection against heart disease and general all round health. They also ensure a healthy circulation and immune system amongst other important functions that are too many to mention here. There is conflicting information however, as to their usefulness in pregnancy. Concern is really over the mercury levels in fatty fish, which is a good dietary source of omega 3 fatty acid. However, given that EFAs are vital to the growing baby (brain & spinal cord development) so it should not be avoided. If concerned, an alternative choice could be to try vegetarian sources (such as flaxseed or hemp seed oil) or take supplements made from algae sources as these pose no dangers for pregnant women. Taking these supplements in moderation is always the sensible approach and if in doubt, it is best to seek advice from a herbalist or a nutritionist.

Other measures for boosting energy include lymphatic drainage (a type of massage that encourages the free flow of lymph fluid through the lymphatic system enabling the efficient removal of toxins and debris from the system). It is a form of enhanced 'detox' so that toxins do not build up in the cells, tissues or surrounding fluids. Diet is also important in general detox as is eating the right kinds of foods for improved nutritional status, boosting circulation (eg. via exercise) and enabling the body to make better use of energy within cells. This requires de-cluttering the system, eliminating toxins, improving current sluggishness of the liver, improving circulation to the cells so oxygen actually reaches the cells for energy production. For general advice on food intake in post-viral fatigue, stress or nervous exhaustion, see under 'Important Aspects of Nutrition' which is discussed later in this chapter.

(ii) Skin, hair, nails and feet

Skin, hair and nails all originate from the same tissue in the skin before they differentiate or specialise into the different structures. Therefore any health advice for maintaining good skin also applies to some extent for hair and nails. The health of the skin is extremely important and as described in earlier chapters, the skin is essentially an organ and must be regarded with the importance that it carries in relation to its many functions.

Many people neglect the skin thinking that it will take care of itself by virtue of a basic skin regime and a passing interest in popping a vitamin pill. However, modern living, a poor lifestyle, environmental hazards, climate change and overexposure to strong sunlight all have a detrimental effect on the skin. Common risk factors include smoking, alcohol, not drinking enough water, a bad diet, a lack of sleep, poor circulation and a poor skincare regime. To appreciate the importance of looking after the skin, it is perhaps best to start at its function and the various constituents that make up this incredible organ.

Skin is made up of water, fat and connective tissue. The latter is made from collagen (which gives the skin its resilience) and elastin, which provides suppleness and youth. With age, the structure of the skin changes and there is loss of integrity in the collagen and elastin which makes the skin appear wrinkled and not so resilient. Therefore great care must be taken to look after it and to protect it. Fat cells are also present underneath the skin and its distribution varies throughout the body. Its purpose is to insulate the body and act as an energy reserve. Fat is essential to the appearance and health of the skin and anyone who is extremely underweight has little fat in their body which seriously compromises the health and function of the skin. Infections, spots, ulcerated wounds and sores are common in skins where there is little fat. Another constituent in the skin is melanin. This is the pigment that is present in all of us and gives the skin its distinctive colour but it also has a more useful purpose in protecting the skin against ultraviolet (UV) light. We all have the same quantity of melanin in our skins but the depth to which they are located in the skin determines the skin colour. Exposure to sunlight will stimulate production of melanin and this is a natural response as this is the body's way of protecting the skin against UV light. The amount of melanin in our skins is a combination of inherited factors and exposure to sunlight. Melanin is most concentrated in moles and freckles.

Other functions of the skin include waterproofing, temperature control and a sense of touch. All of these functions are compromised if the skin is not in good condition or in good health. Indicators of poor skin are varied from its mere appearance to symptoms such as spots & pimples, a dull complexion, dry skin and red or inflamed patches amongst others. Limiting damage is by far the best approach as it is very difficult to avoid the toxic and hazardous environmental risk factors from sun exposure to environmental pollutants that harm our skin.

The following is a general guideline as to the kind of measures that can be adopted to maintain the health & vitality of the skin. This in turn will promote good health of the skin which has many other benefits beyond the visual appearance.

Steps to maintaining good skin:
- Diet & nutritional status
- Lifestyle practices
- Skin products (dispelling common myths)
- Skin hygiene & skincare regimes
- Current concerns with sun-tanning

Diet & nutritional status
To make sure that the skin remains healthy, it is vital to make sure that the diet is good and there is good circulation to the skin surface. Important nutrients include the following:

Nutrient	Comment	Food sources
Protein-rich foods	Cells require protein for growth and repair. The top layer of the skin (epidermis) is effectively dead but the layer just below it is constantly growing and repairing and determines the appearance of the skin at a later stage.	Fish, chicken, eggs, wholegrains, pulses, lean meats,
Antioxidant combo (vitamins A, C and E)	Prevents free radical damage to cells and tissues including the skin. Free radicals are produced through the normal course of metabolism, sometimes to protect the body against viral or bacterial attack. With good nutrition and a healthy immune system, the damage caused by free radicals is prevented or limited. However, through poor diet & lifestyle and a	Citrus fruits, red berries, carrots, wholegrains, green leafy vegetables, broccoli, cabbage, nuts & seeds

	toxic environment, damage caused by free radicals become significant, causing disease (eg. cancer, heart disease) and this accumulates with age.	
B vitamins	These help in the body's metabolic processes, which in turn makes sure that the skin stays smooth and supple. Dry, itchy skin is a common sign of vitamin B deficiency so diet needs to be examined carefully.	Red meat, poultry, fish, eggs, bananas, wholegrains, marmite, brewer's yeast, peanut butter
Essential fatty acids (omega 3 essential fatty acids)	Vital for skin health and appearance. Prevents drying up and promotes proper waterproofing of the skin so that it is not at risk of infection or other skin problems. Good for inflammatory skin conditions as well as dry skin conditions and provides some of the fatty material in the oily secretions of the skin that keep it smooth, supple and waterproof.	Fatty fish (salmon, mackerel, trout, tuna, sardines), walnuts, pumpkin seeds, flaxseeds, flaxseed oil and hemp seed oil
Vitamin E (externally)	An important antioxidant (see above). Good at healing scars and preventing signs of skin ageing.	Fatty fish, wheatgerm, seeds, avocado, almond, sesame oil & green leafy vegetables
Whole food diet	This refers to a diet where no processing has taken place and food is cooked or prepared in its whole form. Mainly fresh ingredients and raw foods that have not been chemically or genetically altered. Whole foods have no additives and preservatives in them. They limit the damage of toxic overload and any potential allergy or reaction to artificial colours or ingredients that could trigger an inflammatory skin reaction or similar.	Nutritionally better for general all round health as it limits the toxic triggers that are the cause of many health problems
Water	Lack of water can leave the skin looking dry, dehydrated and dull in complexion. Water is needed to boost the health of skin cells, helping it shed old cells, keeping it clean and maintaining a healthy glow from skin cells that are moist, plump and hydrated.	Pure water is best, try filtering it first or drink mineral water. Daily quantity should be about 2 litres daily and more for active people

Sulphur	Essential for the production of collagen (component in the skin that makes it resilient) and also helps in healing so particularly good for wounds, acne, inflammatory skin lesions and burns. Vital ingredient in many commercial skin supplement preparations eg. MSM which is taken more for arthritis & other inflammatory joint conditions.	Vegetables (legumes), eggs, fish, onions, garlic
Selenium	An antioxidant – prevents free radical damage	fish, shellfish, red meat, grains, eggs, chicken and garlic. Vegetables can also be a good source if grown in selenium-rich soils.
Prebiotics & Probiotics	Probiotics replenish or top up with friendly bacteria since gut function is vital to good health. A poor digestive system impairs the body in its ability to detoxify harmful substances and toxic build up is reflected in the skin. Prebiotics is the general term given to the raw materials that feed the growth of the friendly bacteria because they won't flourish to healthy numbers if the food supply is low. These food materials are invariably indigestible foods that come from carbohydrate fibres called oligosaccharides. Because we can't digest them, they stay in the gut and stimulate the growth of our friendly bacteria.	High fibre foods, wholegrains, miso, yoghurt, beans, lentils, fruits & vegetables. Good sources of prebiotics include fruits, legumes (eg. pulses, beans, nuts) and wholegrains (eg. wheat, oats, barley, rice)
Herbal skin savers	• Chamomile (externally and internally) for anti-inflammatory action. Soothes and calms irritated skin • Lemon balm, passion flower (tea) – to combat stress which can cause outbreaks in the skin • Comfrey (externally) to heal any skin outbreaks, soothe and reduce inflammation • Aloe vera – great skin moisturiser, heals and soothes irritated or inflamed skin • Centella – good for repairing skin • Witch hazel – an effective astringent so will	Can be individually prepared or combined for a specific purpose. Advice needs to be sought before taking anything internally

	reduce inflammation and redness • Calendula – good for wound healing • Rosewater – natural cleanser and toner. It also stimulates the skin by increasing blood flow to the surface	

Foods to avoid or limit

Food(s)	Comment
Caffeine	Too much stimulants adds to the toxic burden on the system. If the body cannot eliminate these efficiently, it will show in the skin. Best to limit coffee and tea although in moderation, they have other health benefits.
Alcohol	Has a drying effect on the body and depletes vital oils and water from the skin. Makes the skin look dry and flaky. Take in moderation and drink plenty of water to counterbalance the effects of alcohol.
OTC medicines or prescription drugs	If at all possible, avoid resorting to OTC medicines or prescription drugs as a first resort. It is always best to regard them as a last resort or in cases of emergency as far a possible. Try more natural remedies first and explore the reasons and cause of the problem in the first instance.
Fast foods	Full of unhealthy fats and additives that burden the system. Toxic overload will show in the skin which can become prone to outbreaks of spots & pimples, dry, flaky skin and red patches of inflamed skin.
Foods high in refined sugars	Increased levels of blood sugar will increase the risk of infection not only internally but also in the skin. It will aggravate any existing skin disorder or problem so limit or cut out all foods high in refined sugar.
Processed foods & pre-prepared foods	In a similar manner to fast foods, these foods are packed with artificial additives and preservatives which make it harder for the body to process them. There is a risk that the system will become overloaded with toxins. This will at some point be reflected in the skin which will look sallow, dry and lacking in shine or glow.

Lifestyle practices

- Exercise – necessary to improve blood flow to the skin surface. This will ensure that the nutrients for the skin reach the cells and encourage good repair and growth of new cells.
- Smoking – this promotes premature ageing of the skin as the chemicals in cigarettes destroy the connective tissue components in the skin. Loss of elasticity, resilience and premature wrinkle formation are all classic hallmarks of cigarette smoking.

- Alcohol – has a dehydrating effect on all the cells in the body, including the skin. Excessive alcohol makes the skin look dry and lacklustre.
- Diet (see above)

Skin products

- Cleansers – can range from lotions, gels and wipes to simply using soap. Absolutely vital in skin regimes as the dirt and grime need to be removed at the end of the day. This is more important in a climate of increased pollution and if living in busy cities. It is best to stick to a cleansing routine or product that is compatible with skin type and texture rather than trying out new products for the sake of fashion or marketing claims of a 'new and improved' product.
- Moisturisers – absolute must, particularly for older skins. This replenishes the skin of moisture that is slowly depleted from then skin throughout the day. Important to invest in good products that have a sunscreen factor. Lotion is better for the day and a night cream is essential for night time moisturising. Older skins require more care than younger skins although with levels of pollution and environmental toxins aplenty, one is never too young to start a rigorous skin care regime. Again, it is best to stick to something that is tried and tested and is compatible with your skin. By far the best moisturiser is a combination of good diet, lifestyle and an effective skincare regime.
- Exfoliating rubs & treatments – these are designed to remove dead skin cells from the uppermost layer of skin. Normally they slough off at a steady rate but sometimes, they can slow down (many factors affect this) and build up on the skin surface. This gives the skin a dull and lack lustre appearance so exfoliating with a product or simply massaging it with a flannel (face) or a loofah mitt (body) will assist the process. Good moisturising afterwards is essential to prevent the skin from drying out
- Anti-winkle creams – there are many claims made by manufacturers of creams, lotions and gels all of which promote the notion of being able to defy the ageing process. Many of these products are ridiculously expensive and very often unnecessary as no amount of anti-wrinkle remedy will counteract the long-term effects of poor diet, smoking, excessive alcohol intake and sun damage. More fundamental factors beyond the environment such as genetic inheritance have an overriding influence in some people. Time and money is better invested in a more natural approach to healthy skin which incorporates some lifestyle changes and good nutrition as a foundation for limiting the worst effects of ageing.
- Cellulite-busting creams – again, more commercial and marketing hype than actual effectiveness. A more radical examination of society's view on body image and what is considered beautiful and healthy is required. Healthy skin and a healthy body requires discipline, hard work and a dedicated approach to proper nutrition and exercise. No amount of marketing gimmick is going to alter that.

Skin hygiene & skincare regimes

- Cleansing – removes dirt and grime that has built up during the day and must be removed before bedtime

- Moisturising – replenishes important moisture that has been lost throughout the day. Some products also encourage repair and growth of new skin cells
- Exfoliating – removes old skin cells from the surface of the skin which can sometimes remain in the uppermost layer and give the complexion and dull and lacklustre appearance
- Massaging – encourages blood flow to the skin surface so that important nutrients can reach the skin surface. Also encourage repair of damaged skin cells and some massages (eg. lymphatic drainage) actively encourage the removal of toxins and lactic acid build up with has other health benefits in addition to improving the health of the skin
- Cellulite – the term given to the manner in which fat is deposited under the surface of the skin. Characteristic dimpled and 'orange peel' effect is more common in women and in those who have a poor diet, poor skin circulation and those who do not take enough exercise, although this is not always the case. Cellulite is age-related being more common in the older woman. Worst excesses can be offset through regular exercise, limiting caffeine and fast foods and regular massage and skin brushing to promote circulation to the skin
- Nourishing (food) – eating the right foods is vital to healthy skin. See above for recommendations
- Sun exposure – excessive exposure to strong sunlight, particularly without adequate sun protection is disastrous for the skin especially fair skins which are prone to sunburn. The risks for cancer increase in previously sunburnt skins so avoiding this is a sensible precautionary measure.
- Cold weather, wind and rain can also wreak havoc on the skin. Adequate protection with good moisturising properties as well as sun protection (even on grey, dull days, UV damage is still possible).

Current concerns with sun-tanning (sun protection tips)
- Spray tanning – this is a synthetic tan sprayed onto the skin (in a protected environment) and which can last up to a few weeks. This prevents the need to go out and sunbathe with long exposure to sunlight increasing the risk of skin damage and other potential risks. A favourite of many celebrities.
- Suntans – suntans *per se* can look very natural and give a healthy glow to the skin. Exposure to natural sunlight for short bursts every day is a great boost to mood, energy and vitality, particularly if work requirements mean long hours spent indoors. However, many people becomes obsessed with having an all-year tan and this encourages long exposure to sunlight, sometime longer than is advisable or necessary to the point that irreversible damage is done to the skin. If a suntan is a must, it is best to invest in proper, sensible precautions and effective sun protection, although overexposure to sunlight is never going to be beneficial to the skin.
- Skin cancers – there are various skin cancers which are becoming increasingly common. There can be a variety of reasons for this increase including climate change (sunlight is stronger), poor education on the risks of overexposure and inadequate sun protection, genetic risk (inherited factors), smoking, those with fair skins & red hair and those who have a tendency to burn. There are various skin cancers from basal cell skin cancer to squamous cell skin cancer. The most aggressive type though is malignant melanoma although they are less common. It is imperative that all moles on the skin are monitored very carefully (see below).

– Suncreams & sun protection – the most common type of sun protection is to use a sun screen which is found in all sun creams and sun lotions. There are sun protection factors (SPFs) in all these products which is effectively the chemical screen which offers protection from UV light (UVA and UVB light). SPFs can range from 10 to 60. Equally, avoiding the sun between 11am to 3pm (or 10am to 4pm in hotter climates), covering up with suitable clothing, wearing appropriate sunglasses and a wide-brimmed hat is just as important in protecting the skin. Sun creams rub off in water and with time so re-application is essential. After-sun care is also vital, so soothing lotions such as aloe vera gel, lavender gel or a combination chamomile & aloe vera gel will prevent the effects of sunburn and subsequent damage to the skin. Children require extra protection as their skins are very delicate and are easily prone to damage. Sun damage or sun burn at an early age can predispose to cancer in adulthood.

– Monitoring all moles on the skin closely is a prerequisite when sunbathing. Abnormal changes can be a precursor to malignant change. Most skin moles are normal and harmless. However, sometimes they can change in size, shape, colour and manner which can also be harmless. Keeping a close eye on changes is necessary so look out for the following changes and if in doubt, see a doctor:

1. it has changed in appearance
2. it has recently grown or changed shape
3. it has changed colour, varying in shade
4. it has an uneven edge
5. it has become raised or inflamed with a red edge
6. it has started to bleed, ooze or crust
7. it has become bigger than the other moles
8. just looks unusual

Skin through the decades

- 20s – skin may be relatively wrinkle free but this is the decade in which to establish a good skin care regime and to work out the products for cleansing and moisturising. It is also the decade in which to implement dietary and lifestyle practices that are good for the skin.

- 30s – from 30 years onwards, the skin starts to lose tone and muscle mass which can be easily detected in neglected skins. There has to be a greater emphasis on exercise, diet and moisturising as skin can look dry and lacking in shine.

- 40s – the skin has started to thin and an accumulation of environmental toxins, exposure to sunlight and loss of protective function can all be tell-tale signs of age. Moisturisers need to contain chemicals that fight free radicals as the skin becomes drier and tighter with loss of barrier protection against the elements.

- 50s and over – skin shows visible signs of ageing with wrinkles, age spots, brown pigmentation spots and evidence of sun damage. For women, hormonal changes with the menopause also make the skin thinner and drier through lack of oestrogen. Effective moisturising with SPF is essential as is nutrition, particularly antioxidants and intake of sufficient essential fatty acids to combat the effects of an aged skin.

Steps to healthy hair

Hair is essentially dead by the time it leaves the skin surface but the health of the scalp is very important in maintaining healthy hair. It is also important to feed the hair follicles which lie deep below the skin surface as this is very much alive and relies heavily on proper nutrition and a healthy circulation. In short, the health of the hair is dependent on a healthy skin so all the things that apply to skin also apply to hair. The health of the hair is affected a number of factors such as:

1. Diet – vital to the hair follicle from which the hair grows. Poor nutrition will deprive hair of protein, pigmentation, oils and resilience. This can leave the hair shaft prone to breakages, being lacklustre and brittle.

2. Overexposure to strong heat – heat treatments such as blow dying, sun exposure, colour treatments or bleaching, straighteners, tongs, curlers and excessive use of products can all leave the hair shaft dry, brittle, dull and fragile. If heat treatments are to be used, it is advisable to use heat protection products first or limit their use. Towel drying first before any heat treatment is vital and limit making direct contact with heat (hold the dryer at least a few inches away), swap metal plates on straighteners with ceramic ones (less damage) and invest in a good brush. Brush hair nightly to distribute the natural oils throughout the hair before going to bed. A weekly intensive moisture treatment like hot oil is recommended along with good nutrition.

3. Circulation – a poor circulation to the skin can deprive the hair follicle of the essential nutrients for producing a healthy head of hair. Proteins, vitamins, oils and the pigments which give hair its colour all depend of good circulation. Exercise is a great boost to circulation especially to the skin surface. Regular scalp massages can help especially if it is dry and flaky. Oils such as avocado, jojoba or coconut oil are all good choices in nourishing and moisturising a dry scalp.

4. Stress – any stressful factor will limit the flow of blood and the supply of essential nutrients to the skin surface. This will have a negative impact on the hair and it may start to look lifeless, dull, excessively greasy or in contrast, very dry and brittle. Anxiety, worry or shock will temporarily limit blood flow to the roots and hair follicles and reduce the levels of pigmentation. This is perhaps why some may go prematurely grey through excessive worry and anxiety but this is not always the case as there are other overriding factors such as genetic inheritance to consider. In any event, excessive or persistent stress is not a good thing for the hair or indeed the body in general.

5. Extreme weather conditions – cold, wind, rain as well as excessive sun exposure all have a damaging effect on the hair, stripping it if the essential oils and making it appear dull, lifeless, lacklustre and brittle. Good protection and conditioning is vital especially in the winter months as less attention is paid in colder weather conditions.

6. Cleansing regimes - poor hair cleansing regimes will always reveal itself in the appearance of hair. Shampooing and conditioning is a must but more emphasis needs to be placed on conditioners than on shampoos. Frequent washing requires a mild shampoo so that the hair is not stripped of its all important natural oils. Changing conditioners regularly is also needed so that hair can respond better to the treatments. Weekly intense moisture treatments (eg. hot oil wraps) are essential if heat treatments such as blow drying are a part of the styling regime.

Steps to healthy nails

Like the hair, the health of the nails is dependent on a healthy skin. The recommendations for healthy skin as described also holds true to a large extent for healthy nails. Some of the common problems with poor nail health is that they become brittle, breaking off easily, pitting and white spots, sore and red cuticles, dry skin around the edges leading to tears in the skin and nails that look dull and discoloured. The indicators for healthy nails are half moon or crescent moon at the base of the nail, a pink nail bed implying good blood flow to the fingertips, shiny nails, strong nails that do not break easily and a smooth surface that is not ridged, pitted or cracked. The nutritional needs of the nail are as important as the needs of the skin so many of the nutrients required for healthy skin is also necessary for healthy nails. So, protein, B vitamins, sulphur, selenium, antioxidants, essential fatty acids in addition to an overall healthy diet is important. Common problems such as white spots on the nails are due to a zinc deficiency. Taking a zinc supplement (15mg per day) can help in treating it quickly. Thereafter, it is important to get a balanced diet that includes foods that are rich in zinc such as meat, kiwi fruit, shellfish, milk, dairy foods, bread and cereals with wheatgerm.

Other practical measures include:

- Using hand cream regularly – this will prevent dry skin and dry nails. Nails require just as much moisture as skin as they are vulnerable to the elements as the skin and hair. For a weekly moisturising treatment, rinse the hands with warm water then apply generous amounts of a rich hand cream and wear some cotton gloves for a few hours or do this at bedtime.
- Oiling the cuticles – this will prevent splitting of the nails and will give them an added shine. In the long-term, it will make the nails stronger and less prone to breakages.
- Nail regime – this has to be as important as skin regime. Much can be said about a person's nails and a well manicured hand is far more appealing than dirty, scruffy unkempt fingernails. Invest in a good base coat if polish is to be applied. Regular polish is not always good so leave adequate 'breathing space' between applications and scrub the nails with a good nail scrub to remove all traces of old polish that can get embedded in the nail and give a dull appearance.
- Regularly use a nail buffer – this will boost the shine and increase blood flow to the nail surface giving it a better appearance. Apply limited pressure as being too vigorous can thin the nail.
- Always wear washing up gloves when doing the washing.

Steps to healthy feet

Feet are very often neglected and considering the toll that they are put through on a daily basis, it is unsurprising that people suffer from feet problems. There are a variety of common foot disorders; some of these have been discussed in Chapter 4 under the specific conditions. Common examples are athlete's foot and verrucas but there are others such as:

- Corns and calluses
- bunions
- 'hammer toes'
- ankle problems
- in-growing toenails
- fungal infections of the toenails and feet

- dry, cracked soles

Most of these problems can be avoided through basic hygiene and proper care of the feet including wearing sensible footwear (outside of special occasions). Similar to care of the hands, feet require moisturisation, nail care, maintenance and regular 'feet treats' such as massage, pedicure or simply a scented foot soak. The soles of the feet in particular, require extra attention especially in moisturising. The soles of the feet are prone to drying out which leaves them exposed to getting cracked. This in turn leads to skin being broken if it is not addressed promptly. This increases the risk of infection especially if walking barefoot.

Dry skin needs to be repaired, hard skin needs be filed down and footwear needs to be examined and addressed particularly if walking or standing for long hours during the day. Learning to walk properly will prevent further posture-related problems that can affect the feet and wearing the appropriate shoes for back and joint health. If specific help is required, it is best to seek the advice and treatment from a podiatrist or a pedicurist if feet grooming is required.

(iii) Spine and posture

A good posture is dependent on a healthy spine. Many of us take our spine for granted and have acquired some bad habits with posture. As a consequence, injury and illness through these are quite common. Back pain alone costs the UK around £6 million in lost revenue, benefits, treatments and decreased productivity. Current rates put the figure at 2 out of every 5 adults suffering from back pain and whilst a number of cases are from unavoidable causes such as accidents or disease, the majority are essentially from 'wear and tear', poor posture and a lack of sensible precautions such as carrying heavy bags inappropriately or even wearing shoes that are not 'sensible' for the back.

Other examples of the factors that affect the health of the spine:

- Inappropriate footwear especially for walking long distances (lack of appropriate shock absorbers in the shoes can put extra strain on the ankle joints and subsequently the lower back)
- Slouching over a computer screen all day (excessive strain on the spine and the muscles that support it)
- Incorrect posture when sitting or standing (puts extra strain on the spine)
- Lack of exercise (loss of muscle tone & strength that support the spine)
- Exercising without adequate protection for the spine or surrounding structures
- Carrying heavy shoulder bags and other baggage (put an unnecessarily heavy burden on the spine and the strains the muscles that support it). Ruck sacks are better as they distribute the weight more evenly.
- Sleeping without proper support (examine mattress quality; orthopaedic mattresses may be necessary)
- Standing up for most of the day (extra strain on the back and supporting muscles)

The importance of the spine and posture can never be adequately emphasised. The spine supports the entire body, along with the relevant muscles, ligaments, tendons and bone attachments that extend from it. Good health of the spine is important in preventing illness (eg. poor digestive and respiratory function as a result of poor posture) and in preventing injury (eg. muscle strain, wear and tear of joints). Equally, a healthy spine is only as healthy as a good posture. Poise, stance, posture and deportment are all terms used to describe the manner in which the body is held in position when a person stands, walks or moves. This is critical to good health and many of us have a bad posture, possibly acquired through bad habits or through repetitive movements and carrying heavy baggage which can cause excessive pressure on one side of the body causing it to lean in an attempt to accommodate the load. This affects the balance of the body and the spine and supporting structures constantly try to offset any injury by working harder to maintain balance. This can lead to strain and stress on certain structures and possibly injury with time.

A good posture is essential for good health for a number of reasons:

- Can make a person look taller & slimmer
- Improve breathing by increasing lung capacity
- Prevent strain and injury of important structure that support the body (vertebrae, ligaments, muscles & tendons)
- Can prevent slouching
- Can prevent or reduce symptoms of illness in the gut (eg. heartburn caused by slouching, poor digestive function, respiratory disorders and breathing difficulties)

Equally, and often understated, emotions can affect posture and the range of emotions need to be examined carefully in relation to the body's responses to them. For example, when you are stressed or anxious, the body becomes tense and rigid. This causes the muscles in the neck, shoulders and upper back to become tense and this constricts blood flow to that area. In a depressed individual, their body may become slumped and the shoulders may droop which will affect breathing and effective lung function. In the long term, the energy that is used in maintaining these postural distortions will eventually make the body very tired, lethargic and weary.

Important posture-improving techniques:

Alexander technique	Re-learning how to stand, sit and how the body supports itself naturally. Examines the relationship between the head, neck and back, and then all other parts of the body.
Yoga	A series of exercises and body positions that strengthens and tones all parts of the body and is especially good for posture. It strengthens the muscles that support the spine, particularly the lower back and therefore good for alignment.

	Various types of yoga systems are fast becoming popular across gyms and health clubs.
Pilates	A form of exercise that encourages proper alignment of the spine and associated structures. Good for strengthening muscles that support the spine and is very good for posture.
Body balance	An exercise system that, as the term implies balances the body by promoting good alignment and therefore enables good posture.
Exercise eg. swimming	Excellent all round exercise but back stroke is particularly good for supporting the spine. Builds strength, tone, agility, endurance and power. Supporting the muscles of the spine can prevent injury to the back by building strong muscles in that region.
The Feldenkrais method	Similar to the Alexander technique, it re-trains the muscles so that good posture can be achieved. It also encourages good co-ordination so that movement is more agile, graceful and elegant.

(iv) Important aspects of nutrition

There is an awful lot of information about nutrition and diet from magazines, to TV programmes and even specialist programmes dedicated to food and nutritional matters. It is unsurprising therefore that many people remain confused and bewildered by the array of foods and advice that is available. This section of the book does not aim to cover the entire matter on good nutrition as this is beyond the scope of this book, nor does it give specific advice in special cases. It does however provide information on some of the fundamentals on nutrition, something that we have perhaps forgotten with the numerous options on food that are cleverly marketed as being beneficial to the body. It gives a general outline as to the basics on nutrition and what the body actually needs and is designed to process. In this respect, there are important aspects of nutrition that forms the basis for good health and vitality, something that is rarely obtained and adhered to in the fast, frantic pace of modern living.

The basic principle of good nutrition is very much focused on getting a 'balanced diet'. This phrase has been bandied about on many of the consumer programmes and press on matters of health and well-being but what does this actually mean? Simply put, it refers to getting all the correct foods in their right quantities every day. In order to achieve this, it is very important to be familiar with what the correct foods and what the right quantities are. This has been summarised below:

1. Macronutrients	carbohydrates proteins fats
2. Micronutrients	vitamins minerals
3. Fibre (previously called roughage)	
4. Water	

As highlighted, there are 4 aspects to a good diet. Getting all four food substances is vital to good health, well-being and vitality. Ensuring this will also prevent illness and problems that arise due to a lack of them in the diet (dietary deficiencies).

Recommended proportions and choices of foods for a balanced diet

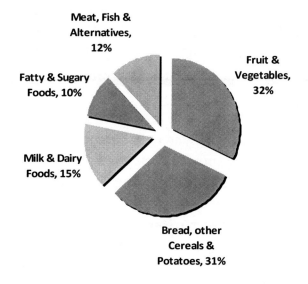

Fruit & Vegetables
Need to aim for 5 portions each day and choose a wide variety of both

Bread, other Cereals & Potatoes
Eat all types and choose high fibre kinds wherever possible

Milk & Dairy Foods
Choose lower fat alternatives

Fatty & Sugary Foods
Try not to eat these too often, and wherever possible, have small amounts

Meat, Fish & Alternatives
Choose lower fat alternatives wherever possible and leaner cuts of meat

The next important aspect is to get the correct proportions of these food substances. Most of us in the West are eating far too much of the fats and carbohydrates and not enough protein, fibre or indeed the micronutrients. Substituting these for supplements is never the long-term solution and is by no means a justification for consuming far too much carbohydrates and fats. Very often, we are told that these are 'wrong foods'. There is no such this as a 'wrong food' unless it is unrecognisable, entirely synthetic or pumped full of additives. In fact carbohydrates and fats are vital to good health and many of us could benefit from re-education about food and re-programming ourselves to choose different foods and to develop ways in which to make them more interesting and tasty. Varying the foods is also good for the body as this will ensure that the right balance of nutrients is obtained. Limiting foods that may trigger illness, allergy or an intolerance are the obvious and sensible measures to adopt in such cases.

Maintaining good health is dependent not only on getting a balanced diet but also in getting the correct proportion of the 4 food categories. In short, more is needed of the macronutrients (carbohydrates, proteins, fats) than the micronutrients (vitamins and minerals). Plenty of fibre needs to be eaten every day as well as plenty of water. Too many of us are not drinking enough water with the consequences of dehydration.

Carbohydrates
There are 2 types of carbohydrates that are important to our health: starch and sugar. Both of these are vital to our health and well-being because they provide energy although we are not eating the right types or quantities of starches or sugars. Aim to have more of the starchy foods such as bread, pasta, potato, rice and cereals. Aim for wholemeal and 'brown' versions which will have more fibre in them than the 'white' versions. These are complex carbohydrates which means that they release sugar slowly into the bloodstream and therefore not overload the system with too much sugar too soon. This is much better for the body. The other type of carbohydrate is sugars and some of them (simple or refined sugars) are far too abundant in the western diet. Natural sugars such as those found in fruits and some vegetables are much better for the body than the refined versions that we see so much of in foods. Avoid foods such as cakes, biscuits, chocolates, sweets and many of the processed or pre-packed foods as they often contain 'hidden sugars'. Other culprits include soft drinks, jam, puddings, pastries and ice cream.

Proteins
Proteins are vital to growth and repair of cells and tissues. These have a limited life span and daily wear and tear requires replenishing of these cells and tissues. Important structures like muscles, tendons, ligaments,

skin, hair and nails all require protein. Key biological compounds such as hormones and other chemical signalling molecules are protein-based. The importance of proteins in our diet cannot therefore be adequately emphasised.

Foods that are good sources of protein include meats, fish, poultry and vegetables. It is preferable to choose lean cuts rather than any other in order to limit the fat intake, particularly saturated fats. Good vegetarian sources include soya beans, seeds, pulses, grains and legumes. A consultation with a nutritionist is highly recommended in the first instance to compile a diet sheet if a radical overhaul of the current diet is necessary.

Fats

There has been much adverse publicity on fats but they are vital to health and well-being. The confusion has arisen due to the type of fats that are consumed and the imbalance in what we eat far too much of. Modern diets contain a disproportionate amount of saturated fats, trans fatty acids and hydrogenated fats. The body requires a certain amount of saturated fats although we are currently eating too much of these. Saturated fats in their natural form are found mainly in animal fat although fried foods also contain a high quantity of these depending on how they are prepared. Trans fatty acids and hydrogenated fats are not found naturally and the body is not designed to process these. As a consequence, they accumulate in the body and can cause ill health through toxic build up. These unhealthy fats are found in most processed foods (eg. biscuits, cakes, crisps, chocolates etc..) and fast foods (eg. take away foods).

In addition to saturated fats (in moderation), other healthy fats are the essential fatty acids (omega 3, 6, and 9) are found in fatty fish and some vegetarian sources such as flaxseeds. This has been discussed earlier in the chapter under Energy.

Vitamins

The best way to get all the necessary vitamins is through food and not from taking a supplement. In cases of deficiency, taking a supplement may be necessary in the short term but this is not the best course of action in the long term. Varying the diet always ensures that the full complement of vitamins is gained through the diet. Important factors such as the quality of the foods purchased, preparation methods, storage and cooking processes must be considered if any vitamin deficiency is to be avoided. The following is a basic summary of the vitamins needed from our diet, their functions and food sources.

Vitamin	Function in the body and/or deficiency disease	Food sources
A (retinol or beta carotene)	Needed for good eyesight, bone formation, gives protection against cancer (antioxidant properties)	Liver, eggs, fresh yellow & red vegetables, broccoli, spinach & most fruits. Food sources need to be fresh to retain optimum levels of vitamin A
B_1 (thiamine)	Supports energy metabolism and nerve function. Deficiency causes beri-beri	Wholegrains, pork, yeast, nuts, dark green leafy (eg. spinach) vegetables, fish & eggs

B_2 (riboflavin)	Supports energy metabolism, normal vision and skin health. Deficiency causes anaemia, dermatitis (skin reactions) and ulceration	Dark green leafy vegetables, mushrooms, eggs, fish and liver
B_3 (niacin)	Supports energy metabolism, skin health, nervous system health and proper digestion. Deficiency causes pellagra or skin disease	Wholegrains, lean meat, fruit, vegetables (eg. spinach), chicken, fish & liver
B_5 (pantothenic acid)	Supports energy metabolism. Deficiency leads to fatigue, headache, cramps & poor circulation	All animal and plant sources especially yeast & eggs
B_6 (pyridoxine)	Protein and fat metabolism, red blood cell production. Deficiency causes anaemia, vomiting and diarrhoea but this is rare	Bananas, watermelon, tomato juice, dark green vegetables (eg. spinach, broccoli), potatoes, squash, rice, chicken
B_{12} (cobalamin)	Needed to make new cells, helps break down fatty acids and amino acids (protein molecules), helps iron absorption, important in immune responses and has antioxidant properties (see below). Stored in the liver & kidneys. Necessary for all cells. Deficiency causes pernicious anaemia and degeneration of nerves and spinal cord	Meats, poultry, fish, milk, eggs & liver
Folic acid (folate)	Needed for the manufacture of the genetic material. Particularly important for pregnant women to prevent birth defects of the fetus	Vegetables such as spinach, sprouts, broccoli, green beans & potatoes. Some bread and breakfast cereals are fortified with folic acid
C (ascorbic acid)	Important for skin health especially collagen synthesis in the skin, amino acid (protein) metabolism helps iron absorption, needed for immunity and has powerful antioxidant properties (see below). Deficiency causes scurvy (skin disease)	Fresh vegetables and fruits (eg. spinach, broccoli, red peppers, tomatoes, kiwi, citrus fruits & strawberries)
D (calciferol)	Promotes bone health. Deficiency in	Made in the skin through

	children causes rickets (abnormal bone development/growth)	exposure to sunlight, milk, eggs, liver, fish
E (tocopherol)	Powerful antioxidant properties (see below) so can help prevent heart disease & cancer. Deficiency in infants can cause brain & spine disorders	Many foods contain vitamin E especially vegetable oils, eggs, liver, wheatgerm, fatty fish, fresh, green leafy vegetables, avocado and milk
H (biotin)	Energy metabolism, fat synthesis, amino acid (protein) metabolism & glycogen (energy reserves) synthesis. Deficiency causes dermatitis (skin reactions) but is rare	All animal and plant sources especially liver, yeast and kidney.
K	Needed for the clotting of blood and the regulation calcium in the blood. Deficiency leads to the risk of haemorrhaging	Brussels sprouts, green leafy vegetables (eg. spinach, broccoli, cabbage) and liver

Minerals

The same principle applies to minerals as to vitamins in that it is always best to acquire these nutrients from the diet rather than through supplementation, although in certain deficiency states, it is best to take supplements in the short term to address the symptoms of deficiency disease. The following is a basic summary of the minerals needed from our diet, their functions and food sources.

Mineral	Function in the body and/or deficiency disease	Food sources
Sodium	Maintains proper balance of fluids and electrolytes. Important for regulating muscle contraction and nerve signalling. Deficiency can lead to muscle cramps, dehydration and poor co-ordination	Salt, soy sauce, bread, milk, meats
Chloride	Important in maintaining balance of electrolytes and helps in digestion	Salt, soy sauce, milk, eggs, fish, meats
Potassium	Maintains proper balance of fluids and electrolytes, cell integrity, muscle contractions and nerve signalling. Deficiency will disrupt all of these functions	Potatoes, spinach, squash, broccoli, avocado, banana, cod, milk
Calcium	Important in health of bones & teeth. Needed for blood clotting process and in	Dairy foods especially cheese & milk, green vegetables

	muscle contraction	
Phosphorus	Important in bone health incl. teeth. Maintains acid-base balance in body systems and is needed in the formation of some important chemicals	Meat, fish, eggs, milk, poultry
Magnesium	Important for bone mineralisation, making of new protein molecules, muscle contraction, immunity and nerve signalling. Deficiency causes muscle cramping, reduced resistance to infection, poor coordination and other biological disturbances	Green vegetables (eg. spinach, broccoli, green beans), tomato juice, pinto beans, black-eyed peas, sunflower seeds, cashews, halibut fish
Iron (Fe)	Formation of haemoglobin pigment in red blood cells. Deficiency causes poor oxygen transport and delivery to cells leading to iron-deficiency anaemia	Liver, artichoke, meat, green vegetables eg. spinach, eggs
Zinc	Important in many enzyme pathways. Needed for wound healing, production of genetic material and proteins, transports vitamin A, needed in sperm production and fetal development. All these functions would be compromised in zinc deficiency states	Oysters, shrimp, crab, meats, spinach, broccoli, green beans
Selenium	A powerful antioxidant. Protects the body against oxidation and therefore offers some protection against disease	Seafood, meats, grains
Iodine	Part of the thyroid hormone (thyroxine) which regulates the metabolic rate (growth & development) of the body	Sea salt, seafood, foods fortified with iodine (eg. cheese, bread, milk)
Copper	Needed for the absorption and use of iron. Important in a number of enzyme pathways and supports haemoglobin (the oxygen-carrying pigment in red blood cells)	Meats
Manganese	Important in many biochemical reactions in the body	Widespread in many foods
Fluoride	Needed for strong tooth enamel and for bone formation	Drinking water with fluorine added, tea, seafood
Chromium	Required for the release of energy (glucose metabolism). Helps normalise blood sugar levels. Deficiency leads to dizziness,	Brewer's yeast, wholemeal bread, rye bread, wholegrains, nuts, cheese and vegetable oils

	irritability, anxiety and sugar cravings	
Molybdenum	Eliminates the products of protein metabolism, strengthens teeth and detoxifies the body from harmful toxins. Deficiency states are not known	Red meats, tomatoes, lentils and beans

Salt

Salt is an important nutrient in our diets because it provides sodium and chloride ions, 2 minerals essential to health and well-being (see above). Unfortunately, we consume far too much of it in our diets because of the amount of fast foods consumed. Additionally, many of the popular convenience foods and pre-prepared foods already have salt in excess of the daily requirement so this further adds to our daily intake. Coupled with the fact we do not drink enough water to balance out the salt intake, it is unsurprising that the Western diet is very unhealthy. One of the main consequences of too much salt intake is high blood pressure. The health risks of high blood pressure (hypertension) have been previously discussed (see Chapter 4).

Fibre

It is certainly the case that the Western diet is unhealthy not least of which is the fact there is very little fibre consumption. The function of fibre is immense and the West is certainly witnessing the health consequences of inadequate fibre in the diet. These range from an increased risk of bowel cancer (possibly others) and diabetes, high cholesterol and obesity through poor regulation of sugar.

Fibre has a crucial function in the body which has not always been noted. Many of the advertising campaigns emphasise the importance of fibre in our diets without fully explaining why. This is because the functions of fibre are diverse but in short, it is essential to good health because it provides bulk to the food, helps flush out toxins from the food and maintains the proper working of the lower bowels which help in eliminating waste products of digestion. In so doing, fibre helps maintain healthy levels of our gut bacteria (the 'good' bacteria), helps keep cholesterol levels in check by trapping some of the substances associated with high cholesterol and regulates sugar release from foods and so can prevent diabetes. Importantly, in having a high fibre diet inadvertently favours a diet that is lower in the refined sugars and fats, both of which contribute to the onset of diabetes.

Dietary fibre is the roughage found in cereals, fruit and vegetables. There are 2 kinds of fibre: water soluble fibre and water insoluble fibre.

- Water-soluble, including pectin, gums, and mucilage. Water-soluble fibre is considered the most health-benefiting type of fibre, especially mucilage fibre
- Water-insoluble, including cellulose, hemicellulose, and lignin

Soluble fibre is found in oats, legumes (peas, kidney beans, lentils), some seeds, brown rice, barley, oats, fruits (such as apples), some green vegetables (such as broccoli) and potatoes. Soluble fibre breaks down as it passes though the digestive tract, resulting in a gel that traps some substances related to high cholesterol.

Evidence exists that soluble fibre may reduce heart disease risks by reducing the absorption of cholesterol into the bloodstream.

Wheat bran and whole grains, as well as the skins of many fruits and vegetables, and seeds, are rich sources of insoluble fibre. The outer fibre layer is often removed in food processing by milling, peeling, boiling or extracting and so people are often not eating enough insoluble fibre. Insoluble fibre makes stools heavier and speeds their passage through the gut. Like a sponge, it absorbs many times its weight in water, swelling up and helping to eliminate faeces and relieve constipation.

Research suggests that 35-50 grams (1-2 ounces) per day brings optimum bowel health for adults, but the average person only gets about 12 grams per day.

High fibre foods include:

- Unprocessed seeds like flaxseeds, psyllium seeds, sesame seeds, sunflower seeds and nuts (but not the oils from them);
- Wheat, oat, barley, and rice bran and other whole grains such as brown rice (but not the white rice or white flour made from them);
- Certain vegetables such as beetroot, asparagus, broccoli, artichokes, carrots, Brussels sprouts, parsnips, spinach, and yams
- Mucilaginous herbs like slippery elm;
- Several kinds of seaweed such as kelp
- Legumes such as kidney beans, pinto beans and soy beans, chickpeas, lentils, and peas;
- Pectin of some fruits such as apples, pears, prunes and raspberries;
- Supplements of concentrated fibre.

Water
Although water has no nutritional value, it is essential to health. Water makes up more than two thirds of the weight of the human body, and without it, humans would die in a few days. We are not drinking enough water and many of us are in fact in a state of perpetual dehydration. Signs of dehydration include fuzzy short-term memory, trouble with basic arithmetic, and difficulty focusing on smaller print, such as a computer screen. Mild dehydration causes fatigue and lethargy.

Water is important to the mechanics of the human body. The body cannot work without it. On a cellular level, all the biochemical processes in the body depend on a level of hydration in the cells, without which they are compromised resulting in the ensuing health risks. In summary, water has the following functions in the body:

- Water serves as a lubricant
- Water forms the base for saliva
- Water forms the fluids that surround the joints.

- Water regulates the body temperature, as the cooling and heating is distributed through perspiration.
- Water helps to alleviate constipation by moving food through the intestinal tract and thereby eliminating waste; water is the best detoxifying agent.
- Regulates metabolism
- Plays a key role in preventing disease by keeping all cells hydrated

Top 10 tips to healthy eating:

1. Limit saturated fat intake and cut out foods with trans fats and hydrogenated fats
2. Increase intake of wholefoods, cereals and wholegrains
3. Eat more fresh fruits and vegetables, organic wherever possible
4. Eat more lean meats than fattier cuts of meat, more fatty fish, poultry or vegetarian alternatives
5. Increase fibre intake
6. Choose reduced-fat dairy products or non-dairy alternatives
7. Limit alcohol intake to celebrations/special occasions
8. Drink plenty of water
9. Limit foods with refined sugars as far as possible & switch to natural sugars and brown sugar if absolutely necessary
10. Limit salt intake as much as possible

General dietary advice in post-viral fatigue, stress or nervous exhaustion

1. Examine protein intake (protein stores may be depleted)
   - pulses, beans
   - wholegrains, soy protein
   - nuts, seeds (flaxseed/linseed, pumpkin seeds, walnuts, sesame seeds)
   - fatty fish (salmon, tuna, mackerel, sardines) at least 3 times/week

2. Examine essential fatty acid intake especially omega 3
   - EPA = eicosapentaenoic acid & DHA = docosahexaenoic acid (fatty fish, nuts, seeds at least 3 times/week)

3. Examine fluid & electrolyte balance
   - Get a juicer (short-term use only), drink plenty of water, green tea/herbal teas instead of coffee and black tea.
   - Make an isotonic drink for short term treatment by mixing 1 teaspoon of sugar & 1 teaspoon of salt in water or diluted fruit juice

4. Examine micronutrient intake
   - Vitamin B supplement
   - Zinc (boosts immune responses)
   - Antioxidants (Vitamins A, C, E and selenium, green tea, bioflavonoids, pycnogenols – pine bark and grape seed extract)

- Iron (leafy green vegetables, red meats, wholemeal bread, dried fruit, pulses). To increase absorption of iron, eat with foods that are rich in vitamin C
- Vitamin B_{12} (dairy products, eggs, cereals with added Vit B_{12}, soya milk)
- Calcium (leafy green vegetables, dairy products, almonds, sesame seeds, dried fruit, foods with added calcium)

5. Food alternatives
   - Organic chocolate instead of non-organic
   - Crush a few fenugreek seeds (*Trigonella foenum-graecum*) and make a tea using the seeds – helps to control sugar cravings

6. Healthier options for nibbles/snacks
   - Dried fruit (for chocolate and sugar cravings). Limit these as they are high in calories as they are concentrated in natural sugars
   - Pumpkin seeds and pine nuts – very tasty and much healthier than crisps
   - Fresh fruit – always the better option especially in their whole form as this will include fibre intake
   - Houmous – low fat options also available. Good on oat cakes or rye crispbreads. Sugar-free and gluten-free alternatives also available
   - Salad – try different leaves and combinations. Add nuts, seeds, flaxseeds and low fat dressings. Vary and experiment. Full of nutrients and fibre. Choose dark green leaves, red, orange or yellow peppers, cous cous, beans or rice.
   - Munch on carrots – very nutritious and very filling
   - Popcorn – high in fibre

7. Quick fixes
   - Bananas (high in energy, good source of potassium and far healthier than chocolate)
   - Avocados (in moderation if watching cholesterol levels but an excellent all-round nutrient - have once/week)

8. Cereal alternatives
   - Porridge oats with grated apple and sprinkle flaxseeds on top for a crunchy texture (benefits include reducing cholesterol, packed with many nutrients, flaxseeds provide omega 3 EFA and fibre, energy booster)

Importance of antioxidants

The ageing process, toxic living, an unhealthy diet and a poor lifestyle all contribute to oxidative stress which produces free radical damage to cells and tissues. Antioxidants are natural chemicals invariably food substances/nutrients which counteract the effects of free radicals and so help reduce some of the damage caused by them. This includes the prevention of disease and some of the age-related symptoms such as arthritic pain, inflammation and cell & tissue degradation. On an another level, antioxidants are thought to confer protection against some of the more serious diseases such as cancer, heart disease, inflammatory disease (eg. ulcerative colitis, arthritis) and possibly some of the more degenerative diseases such as Alzheimer's disease.

A number of food substances have antioxidant properties. Notably, these include, Vitamins, A, C and E. It also includes the mineral selenium but some foods contains naturally high quantities of flavonoids which also have antioxidant properties. Some commercial preparations refer to them as bioflavonoids but essentially they are the same.

Good food sources of antioxidants include the red berries, cereals, and a variety of vegetables. There is a suggestion that eating whole foods has additional benefits when it comes to antioxidants since a combined effect is better than individual antioxidant supplements. Other food sources include legumes, seeds (eg. sunflower seeds) and nuts (eg. walnuts).

1. **Vitamin A** – liver, fish, liver oil, eggs

2. **Beta-carotene** (from vitamin A) – yellow/orange vegetables (eg. carrots, sweet potatoes, pumpkin), yellow/orange fruit (eg. apricots, mangoes, papaya, peaches, oranges)

3. **Vitamin E** – vegetable oils, nuts, wheatgerm, olives, margarine, milk

4. **Vitamin C** – fruits especially citrus fruis eg. strawberries, kiwi. Vegetables eg. red & green peppers, broccoli, Brussel sprouts, tomatoes, potatoes

5. **Selenium** – Brazil nuts, seafood, liver, grains & seeds grown in selenium-rich soil

6. **Pycnogenol** – pine bark and grape seed extract. Found to be 50 times more effective in eliminating free radicals than vitamin E and 20 times more effective than vitamin C.

Other sources of antioxidants:

Antioxidant	Good sources
Berries	bilberry, blueberry, blackcurrant, cherry, strawberry, cranberry, raspberry
Fruit	grape, pomegranate, pineapple, orange, plum, lemon, grapefruit, kiwi, dates, clementine
Legumes	broad beans, pinto beans, ground nut, soy beans
Nuts, seeds & dried fruit	walnuts, sunflower seeds, apricots, prunes
Vegetables	cabbage, kale, peppers, chillies, spinach, Brussel sprouts, artichoke, parsley
Cereals	barley, millet, oats, corn

Maintaining a healthy weight (BMI ratio)

Food labelling practices have changed over the past few years and it is much easier to monitor the quality and quantity of what we consume. With an increasing incidence of clinical obesity affecting many of the industrialised nations, it is becoming ever more important to keep a healthy body weight in order to prevent some of the more chronic and insidious health problems that accompany obesity.

The traffic light system that is currently in use in many food stores across the UK gives an indication of the food content in terms of carbohydrates, proteins, types and quantities of fat, vitamins, minerals, fibre and energy. Of course without the necessary information as to what constitutes the right quantities and what is considered 'bad' for the body, no system of food labelling is going to achieve any benefit to consumers. Education is vital as is proper advice and guidance from trained professionals who provide the necessary information and advice for each circumstance and with consideration of factors such as food intolerances, medical states, disorders, special diets, age and gender. Nutritionists and herbalists often work together to provide the best and most comprehensive advice to consumers who may require some initial guidance, particularly in weight loss regimes and in re-programming themselves to eat more healthily.

The standard that is used to give an indication of normal weight is called the BMI. This stands for the Body Mass Index and is calculated from the person's weight (in kilograms) and a square of their height (in metres). It is a ratio of how heavy a person weighs according to their height.

$$BMI = \frac{weight\ (kg)}{height^2\ (m^2)}$$

BMI Categories:

- Underweight = less than 18.5
- Normal weight = between 18.5-24.9
- Overweight = between 25-29.9
- Obese = BMI of 30 or greater

Recent categories include:

- Clinically Obese = between 30-39.9
- Morbidly Obese = 40 and above

To maintain a healthy weight is essential to good health although this needs to be balanced with proper nutrition and getting the right quantities of all the nutrients. It goes without saying that varying the diet and eating the correct foods, indulging in 'bad' foods in moderation and exercising regularly will automatically keep the body weight in check. Applying this principle as early as possible is advised as this will prevent many of the diet-related problems later on in life.

CHAPTER 6 – TOPICS OF SPECIAL INTEREST

(i) Topics of special interest

Herbs and cancer

It is without doubt cancer remains one of the biggest, most important diseases of the 21st century and whilst significant advances have been made in the treatment and management of this devastating disease, modern medicine is no further forward in finding an effective cure. Many have questioned modern lifestyles including diet and the impact of stress. This is in direct response to the fact that many of the cancers are on the increase and whilst many inherent things about the human body remain fundamentally unchanged, there are many contributory factors and patterns of working and living that have significantly changed. Establishing a conclusive link between modern living, modern diets, modern medicine, environmental and lifestyle factors continue to elude scientists partly because it is difficult to prove cause and effect in any given population and given the genetic variation and individual differences of human beings, more difficult to assess risk factors. Cross-cultural studies may provide more clues as patterns and trends may be easier to detect but it is going to require much more research and analysis.

With regard to cancer, herbal medicine falls into the broad category of natural therapies that have shown great promise and have helped numerous patients. Some of the natural therapies have proved highly controversial simply due to the lack of evidence or proof of their effectiveness, yet patient testimonials and reports of improvement or indeed recovery remains a mystery. Western medical herbalists are trained to refer patients for conventional treatment and management where there is sufficient cause for concern following consultation and/or physical examination. They cannot treat or recommend any form of treatment that falls outside conventional medicine. This is not to say that herbal medicine has no place in the treatment and management of cancer. On the contrary, herbal medicine has much to offer.

Broadly speaking, the rationale within which herbal medicine focuses is on the following:

- Herbs that **prevent** cancer
- Herbs that **stop** the growth of cancer
- Adjunct therapy and management of cancer (supportive role of the herbalist)
- Herbal management of the physical and psychological side effects of cancer treatment
- Palliative care and pain relief

To discuss the therapeutic interventions and the benefits of plant remedies in cancer in any significant detail is beyond the scope of this book. However, the basic strategy can be summarised as follows:

A) Herbalists' Perspective - Building natural defences (which are weakened in cancer onset)

B) Treatment Rationale - To control the cancer without weakening the patient. The following are examined:

- Diet/ Nutritional status
- Emotional aspects in the patient
- Psychological aspects in the patient
- Stress
- Resistance to infection/ Immunity

- to help the body heal itself and fight/ resist disease (cancer) by itself

- adjunct therapy (on the basis that cancer is not only a local disease but a reduction in the body's resistance being the primary cause)

C) Main therapeutic actions of herbal medicine - Boosting vitality

- Immune support

- Liver support

- ↓ inflammation

D) Additional benefits of herbal supplementation

- ↓ toxic effects of chemotherapy & radiotherapy treatments
- ↓ side effects of chemotherapy & radiotherapy
- ↑ sensitivity of conventional treatments for cancer (chemotherapy & radiotherapy)

E) Major considerations in treating a cancer patient

Strengthen body resistance & enhance vitality

- Korean or Siberian ginseng
- Indian ginseng

Immune-enhancing therapy

- echinacea
- astragalus

Removal of blood-stagnation & improve lymphatic drainage

- poke root
- marigold

Detoxification Therapy

- dandelion
- yellow dock
- blue flag

Anti-Inflammatory Therapy

- licorice
- ginkgo

Antioxidant Herbs

- various red-berried fruits & those high in flavonoids eg. bilberry, hawthorn, ginkgo
- grape seed extract

Liver detoxification

- importance of Phase I and Phase II metabolism
- milk thistle
- turmeric
- schisandra
- the brassicas (broccoli, cabbage, horse radish, brussel sprouts…)
- garlic
- rosemary
- sage
- parsley leaf oil
- citrus fruit oil
- green tea

Stress and Psychoneuroimmunology (PNI)

1. the mind-body link is always considered
2. treatment rationale is based within a holistic context/ framework
3. St. John's Wort for depression, anxiety, antiviral, anti-inflammatory action
4. Indian ginseng – stress-busting, nervine tonic, relaxant, mildly sedating
5. valerian – anxiolytic, relaxant, antispasmodic

ORGAN-SPECIFIC APPROACH	*SYMPTOMATIC APPROACH*
Depending on the site of the tumour or body systems under stress, normal, healthy cells are supported, diminish their damage and create an environment for cancer cells to be regulated 1. Liver – milk thistle 2. Mucous membranes – goldenseal 3. Connective tissue restorative – centella	**Pain** – corydalis, cramp bark, valerian **Nausea** – ginger, chamomile, mint **Constipation** – cascara, senna **Diarrhoea** – agrimony, bilberry, oak & other

4. Kidney/Adrenal Support –Rehmannia 5. Brain – bacopa 6. Circulation – ginkgo 7. Breast – poke root 8. Exocrine Pancreas - gymnema, bitter herbs eg wormwood	herbs with a high tannin content **Depression** – *St John's Wort,* damiana, rosehips **Mouth Ulcers** – propolis (topically), centella, goldenseal

Additional Points for Consideration in Management

- dietary considerations (eg. ↓ fat, radical diets)
- antioxidant vitamins (vitamins A, C and E) plus selenium
- soy (xref. Chapter 4 on menopausal symptoms - information sheet on phytooestrogens). Not be taken in oestrogen-dependent cancers such as breast cancer
- herbal intervention (especially as adjunct therapy)
- other natural products (eg. PC-SPES, a blend of 8 herbs taken as a supplement to keep the prostate gland healthy)
- acupuncture (esp. in pain management)
- massage
- exercise
- psychological intervention (counselling, support)
- mind-body interventions (PNI)
- concept of Integrative Medicine

Anti-cancer herbs of likely benefit

- milk thistle – protects the liver
- Siberian ginseng – helps body cope with stress, immune stimulant, cancer protective, ↓ radiation damage to healthy cells & tissues
- aloe vera gel – internally & externally protective
- astragalus & echinacea – supports white blood cell count, helps reduce opportunistic infections
- schisandra – protects the liver, helps body cope with stress and supports the nervous system

HERBAL SUPPORT IN CANCER TREATMENT

A variety of herbal remedies can offer much support during cancer treatment. Supportive therapy through herbal supplementation can address the often distressing, physical side-effects (SE) experienced from radiotherapy and chemotherapy. Additionally, psychological symptoms and the emotional aspects of patient care can be effectively treated with nervines, tonics and adaptogens. Herbal supplementation may help to reduce much of the morbidity associated with cancer therapy since the poor selectivity of presently available anti-cancer drugs make it impossible to avoid some damage to healthy tissues, resulting in the common SE seen within clinical management.

Radiotherapy

Radiation 'cooks cells' in much the same way that microwaves do – healthy cells can also be affected.

- To minimise radiation sickness and nausea
  - kelp metabolises support & protection from tissue damage
  - yarrow as a nervous system and circulatory tonic
  - tree of life as an anti-microbial to combat opportunistic infections
  - apples have valuable anti-radiation properties

- To control nausea
  - ginger
  - fennel
  - dandelion root

- Treatment of burning sensations internally & externally
  - sage has astringent properties
  - comfrey as a vulnerary, demulcent & emollient
  -aloe vera gel is soothing & cooling

- Support liver function
  - milk thistle
  - dandelion leaf & root

- Protection from stroke
  - ginkgo
  - greater periwinkle
  - mistletoe
  - hawthorn

- Immune system support & cancer prevention
  -The ginsengs & goldenseal for general support
  -Aloes – bowel
  - oats – small bowel
  - echinacea – lymph
  - licorice – adrenal

Chemotherapy

- chamomile – gut & nervous system
- milk thistle – liver
- alfalfa – gut
- rosehips – kidney, liver, adrenals, nervous system (antioxidant, iron, vit C)
- tree of life – antineoplastic, astringent, antimicrobial
- parsley – nutrient, iron & other minerals, Vit C

- fennel – pancreatic tonic
- blue flag – thyroid (metabolic regulator)
- ginger – metabolic tonic for toxic shock
- licorice – recovery after severe adrenal shock (also increasing the palatability of herbal prescriptions and therefore compliance)

Additionally: -**Colloidal Silver** has antimicrobial properties however, caution needs to be exercised with this supplement.

-**Garlic and MRSA** : there is some evidence to suggest that garlic can serve a useful purpose in protecting the body against hospital acquired infections such as MRSA and so may be useful for patients during periods of hospitalisation to prevent such infections.

Common side effects & symptoms associated with the cancer itself or in treatment

1. Vomiting – black horehound is an anti-emetic
2. Nausea – ginger
3. Loss of hair/alopecia – vitamin B supplementation
4. Shortness of breath – ephedra, lobelia (prescribed from herbalists only)
5. Persistent fatigue – the ginsengs, astragalus
6. Anaemia (iron deficiency) – nettle leaf, gentian
7. Increased susceptibility to infection – wild indigo, echinacea, garlic
8. Constipation – senna, cascara
9. Diarrhoea – bilberry, walnut
10. Insomnia / poor sleep pattern – valerian, Californian poppy
11. Psychological Symptoms eg. worry, anxiety, depression – range of nervines
12. Weight Loss/ Cachexia – range of bitter herbs eg. wormwood, gentian
13. Altered Growth – possibly metabolic (thyroid) regulators
14. Impaired Fertility – possibly hormone balancers, reproductive system tonics
15. Secondary malignancy – the ginsengs & other immune boosters, lymphatics & alteratives (prophylactic)
16. Mouth ulceration – sage, witch hazel with myrrh as a mouthwash (topically)

HERBAL SUPPORT IN PALLIATIVE CARE

The role of the medical herbalist within palliative care can offer much in respect of symptomatic relief as well as psychological support that is essential within cancer management. Addressing other problems that arise during treatment can ease much of the suffering during the terminal phase of life, making it less traumatic for patients and their families.

A range of nervines can address symptoms such as depression, insomnia, irritability, anxiety etc….. Equally, pain relief can be sought with effective analgesics but requires much liaison between herbalists and the patients' doctors.

Appropriate nutritional advice can be given in order to ensure adequate intakes and to prevent complications arising that can exacerbate or aggravate symptoms.

The advanced stages of palliative care may involve respiratory symptoms and significant pain that can only really be addressed in a symptomatic manner. Much liaison is required here.

PLANTS AND CANCER PREVENTION

Preventative treatment in herbal medicine is essentially to support a patient with a strong familial history of cancer or preventing the reoccurrence of it. Much research is being conducted on plant remedies and indeed many of the conventional drugs currently used with cancer management have some origin or basis in plant medicines.

The American National Cancer Institute (NCI) identified a range of foods with cancer preventive properties. This was very much based on *in vitro* and *in vivo* studies in addition to significant epidemiological evidence. The NCI grouped their research findings into 3 categories:

1.Highest anti-cancer activity found in:

- Garlic -allyl sulfides (active constituents) has numerous health enhancing properties
  -could also ↓ the mutagenic effects of chemotherapy (Chinese research)
  -shown to have some effect against MRSA (more recent UK research)
  -has high levels of selenium (Se), an antioxidant
- Soy beans -contains lignans & isoflavones (phytooestrogens)
- *Ginger*
- Licorice
- Umbelliferous Vegetables eg. carrots, celery, parsley, parsnips (all contain polyacetylenes)

2. Moderate anti-cancer activity found in:

- Onions – contain ally sulphides (numerous health-enhancing properties)
- Linseed (flaxseed) -high in Omega 3 EFA (EPA and DHA) and lignans
- Citus fruits – high in flavonoids
- Turmeric
- Cruciferous vegetables (Brassicas) -broccoli, brussel sprouts, cabbage, cauliflower
  -some animal experiments sugest that these vegs ↑ the metabolism & excretion of oestrogen which could be beneficial in conferring protection against some oestrogen-dependent cancers esp. breast, uterine cancers
- Solanaceous vegetables eg. tomatoes, peppers (contain lycopene)
- Brown rice
- Whole wheat

PROTECTIVE FOODS Some additional & general recommendations

- At least one vegetable in the cabbage family eg. broccoli, cabbage
- Some garlic or onion daily (anti-cancer, lipid-lowering properties)
- Fresh, whole fruits and vegetables
- Antioxidants:

a) combat free radicals that cause oxidative damage that's linked to disease

b) consume foods high in flavonoids

c) vitamins A, C and E, beta-carotene, Se all known to:

- o block various phases of cancer development
- o act synergistically with each other & with dietary components to exert a protective effect
- o main protective effects occur during the 'initiation' and 'activation' phases of cellular change (ie. protects individual groups of cells from carcinogenesis which have bypassed the body's inherent defence systems & mechanisms)

- Recurring suggestion that foods contain many different protective compounds which play an important role – it is vegetables in their entirety, rather than individual components that are protective
- It is advisable that both fruit and vegetables are consumed in their recommended proportions. Fruits should not replace vegetable-filled meals since they are generally lower in minerals and higher in sugars than vegetables and are best consumed whole (not juiced) in order to retain the fibre and slow the absorption rate of sugars.
- Another consideration = Raw vs Cooked
- Carotenoids – red, yellow & orange vegs & fruits (high in beta-carotene = a major antioxidant & cancer preventive food component that is a precursor to Vit A). Significant quantities found in carrots, sweet potato, pumpkin, papaya (paw paw), oranges, apricots, peaches. Also found in dark green, leafy vegetables.
- Lycopene – found in tomatoes
- Beetroot – rec. 200-250g of finely grated beetroot daily. Found to stop the progression of cancer (in most cases) but the mechanism of its action is unknown
- Citrus fruits – Vit C and pectin have been implicated in conferring protection
- Soya products – xref. phyto-oestrogens table in Chapter 4
- Green tea – contain polyphenols with powerful antioxidant properties
- Fibre

a)↓ risk of colon cancer

b)↑ production of short-chain fatty acids which protect the bowel wall from abnormal cell change

c) especially important for women - ↓ risk of oestrogen-dependent cancers incl. breast cancer

d) different types of fibres – ensure adequate intakes of all by incorporating a varied diet and foods in their whole form

- Wheat & Psyllium (husks) – combined is better than each on their own
- Yoghurt & Fermented Milk products – some evidence that bacteria normally in these foods can inactivate carcinogens especially in the bowel. Also implicated in preventing breast cancer

- Foods to reduce or avoid:
    Fats esp. saturated
    Alcohol (but moderate amounts of red wine can be beneficial in other disease)
    Coffee – linked to bladder cancer but paradoxically can ↓ risk of bowel cancer

General Advice: to moderate and vary everything regarding diet.

SUMMARY

- Herbalists' perspective on cancer – onset & treatment rationale
- No herbal treatment can claim to cure cancer
- Herb-drug interactions – can often limit adjunct therapy or progress in management
- Individual differences have to be considered when devising a treatment regimen and must be accounted for. This cannot always be predicted in any given treatment regime
- Importance of diet must be given due emphasis
- Claims by manufacturers of commercial preparations – must be viewed with some caution as they can vary significantly in content, quality, strength & therapeutic efficacy
- Always seek professional help before self-medicating on any herbal medicine.

Without a doubt cancer is big business. And although there is no conventional drug or alternative treatment at present that can reliably claim to cure cancer, there is considerable anecdotal evidence and supportive scientific data to suggest that complementary therapies, particularly herbal remedies, can contribute to cancer prevention, control and reduction in the risk of recurrence.

The strongest scientific evidence supports the value of psychosocial interventions in quality of life and possibly increased life expectancy. In the end it is clear that natural anti-cancer therapies remain unproven as a direct consequence of the lack of research on these agents. It is not that they have been proved useless, it is merely that evidence is lacking to decide one way or the other.

It could be argued that in successful cases where alternative therapies were sought and applied in favour of conventional treatments, the cancer may have reached its natural plateau and sometimes would have abated and resolved eventually. Without a proper study into this however, it would be impossible to comment categorically on the beneficial effects (if any) on popular alternative remedies and treatments. Equally it would be irresponsible to dismiss the large body of anecdotal evidence that exists on their therapeutic efficacy especially when patients have reached the point of desperation and despair.

Until science can firmly establish incontrovertible evidence that natural therapies are ineffective for cancer and, at worst, harmful, it is not in the best interest of all patients and their healthcare practitioners to dismiss claims of therapeutic benefits, even if it does not conform to scientific convention.

Weight loss and herbal medicines

With so many news reports of a global obesity crisis and the numerous warnings and increased awareness of the dangers of excess weight, it is unsurprising that many people have resorted to drastic measures to alleviate some of their concerns. Obesity has now surpassed alcohol as the single biggest cause of liver cirrhosis not to mention the other health risks that obesity poses. The many strategies and measures that people adopt in their attempt to lose weight can range from special diets and exercise to drugs or even surgery. Many have resorted to popping a pill and there are a number of untested substances that manufacturers falsely claim to lose weight. This may pose dangerous consequences for the unsuspecting public who can readily purchase harmful substances claiming to lose weight without getting proper advice from qualified and regulated practitioners such as medical herbalists and nutritionists.

Weight loss can be a potentially complex topic especially as the constitution of each person varies and what works well in one individual may not work so well in another. However, in almost all cases the cause is the same; too much food is eaten for the amount of work being done. There is only an extremely small percentage of the population that have a genuine and real metabolic or 'glandular' problem or even a genetic disorder that can be attributed to excessive weight gain. Getting people to change dietary habits is fast becoming a huge challenge for nutritionists, dieticians and other health care practitioners involved in the concerted effort to reduce the incidence of obesity in the population. It is becoming clear that re-programming individuals and educating the public on food and nutrition, in addition to changing policy on food manufacturing and availability is the only long-term solution to rectifying this global obesity problem.

Herbal medicines by themselves will not enable the body to lose weight. Herbalists prescribe remedies as part of a holistic approach and will recommend lifestyle and dietary changes which will be far more effective in weight loss than any herbal medicine alone. In some instances, prescribing a course of herbs will improve functions of certain organs that will assist in weight loss such as the liver, the kidneys and the circulation. Combined with proper advice about healthy eating and exercise regimes, weight loss in patients is far more effective and long-term than radical diets or taking herbs indiscriminately.

The following gives some information about some of the herbs that may be useful and some that have had much press attention and commercially marketed worldwide.

Herbal Formulas:

Commercial herbal formulas usually contain a combination of herbs that have desirable effects in weight loss such as increasing the metabolism (called thermogenesis), water loss (diuretic effect), increased circulation, boosting energy, increasing bowel movement (laxative effect) and appetite suppression. Thermogenesis is quite literally the generation of heat and can be artificially achieved by taking herbs that increase the thyroid gland (this gland controls the resting metabolic rate), taking stimulants in general like caffeine or ephedra, boosting circulation by taking cayenne pepper or ginger can often achieve this. However, ephedra is not available over the counter (OTC) as it has potentially dangerous effects if taken without proper consultation from a registered herbalist. It is for this very reason that ephedra is not for sale OTC in the UK or the US so purchasing it online or from other non-regulated sources is potentially unsafe. Interestingly though, the main active ingredient in this herb (ephedrine) can be sold OTC and can be found in many of the pharmaceutical preparations such as nasal decongestants. Thermogenesis is often referred to as fat burning but herbs that generally stimulate body systems and improve circulation will undoubtedly burn fat in the course of energy release. It is upon this basis that many of the herbs that stimulate and increase metabolism are popular with dieters. The following describes some of the actions of the herbs often used either as single or combination preparations.

- **Metabolic stimulants**

    As the term implies, these herbs stimulate the metabolic system, that is, they speed up the rate at which energy is released so less fat is stored. The metabolic rate can be at the heart of any weight gain since it declines with age and can become sluggish due to a sedentary, modern lifestyle, a poor diet and lack of exercise. Some herbs increase the metabolic rate and can make better use of the food we eat but to gain full benefit from herbal supplementation, it must be addressed as part of a general overhaul which examines diet and lifestyle in some detail.

    Popular and common herbal stimulants include the ginsengs (Siberian and Korean), caffeine (found notably in coffee and tea but also present in some cocoa, chocolate and some fizzy drinks), ephedra and guarana. It is strongly recommended that a consultation with a medical herbalist is sought prior to any self-medication as some of these herbs can pose serious health risks in some individuals. This is particularly true of ephedra which is not available over the counter in any health food store in the UK. However, there are many unlicenced and unregulated products containing ephedra which can be obtained via the internet and must always be viewed with caution. Although an effective bronchodilator and particularly useful in cases such as asthma, ephedra should not be taken by anyone with conditions such as high blood pressure, heart disease or glaucoma (amongst many other conditions) Side effects can include restlessness, insomnia and tremors. It can also induce high blood pressure in some cases. It is for this very reason that only qualified medical herbalists are licenced to dispense ephedra. Another popular herb is Guarana which is a stimulant made from the seeds of a vine found in Brazil and the jungles of the Amazon. It is popular because it has a flavour similar to chocolate and so it is used in many of their foods and drinks. The Food & Drugs Administration (FDA) in the US has approved guarana as a food additive and it can be found in soft drinks, sweets, drink mixers and weight-loss pills. The caffeine levels found in guarana are stronger than those in coffee or tea and it is therefore harnessed for its stimulating properties. Taken orally as an extract, guarana curbs the appetite and excites the nervous system. These qualities have led companies to include guarana in diet and weight-loss pills which help people keep energy levels up while not eating. It is important to remember that the long-term effects or excessive consumption of any stimulant is not good for the body as it becomes increasingly reliant on it and does not encourage the body to make more efficient use of food or increase the metabolic rate through natural methods such as exercise.

    Another popular herb is kelp (seaweed) which is a natural thyroid stimulant and this may boost the metabolic rate in sluggish systems. Effectively, this boosts the rate at which energy is released from food and reduces the body's desire to store unwanted food reserves.

    Other notable stimulants include green tea, damiana and yerbe mate but proper advice should be sought before taking any herbs. Herbs can be extremely useful in any weight loss regime only with proper care and advice. They cannot exert their full effect by themselves with little change to poor diet and lifestyle choices.

- **Circulatory stimulants**

It is pretty much everyone's experience that eating anything with chillies (cayenne pepper or capsicum) has the effect of increasing the heart rate encouraging sweating and increasing core body temperature. This has the effect of boosting energy release from food and therefore boosting the metabolic rate. Additionally, cayenne has other benefits such as stimulating digestion, improving the immune system and increasing fat burning (thermogenesis). Another circulatory stimulant is ginger and again, in a similar manner increases body temperature. Both herbs have very little impact on weight loss being more effective in the whole process of aiding digestion. Both contain active ingredients that support and stimulate digestion in addition to boosting circulation. In effect, they are more likely to benefit the body by improving the delivery of nutrients to cells and make better use of food through an improved digestive function. In the long-term, this may prevent overeating and regulate body weight through proper use of food.

- **Laxatives**

Many people who diet regularly, use and sometime misuse laxatives in the mistaken notion that this will prevent the body from gaining weight. What this does is to mistreat the body and to encourage the bowels to become heavily reliant on laxatives. This is one of the reasons why herbalists rarely prescribe herbal laxatives on any long-term basis preferring to use it sparingly in the first instance introducing dietary changes that train the lower gut to become more active and also in severe cases where it is absolutely necessary to get things moving. The consequences of constipation and reduced bowel emptying have already been discussed. The build up of toxins due to sluggish bowel movement can sometimes result in weight gain but the use of laxatives is never the answer to weight loss either in the short-term or long-term.

Herbal laxatives fall into 2 categories: those that provide bulk to the food eaten and therefore making it easier for the bowels to work properly and those that increase gut motility so that the transit of food is quicker. Bulk laxatives are the preferred favourite of herbalists and encourages patients to introduce fibre to their diet and to retrain their bowels into functioning more effectively. Good bulk laxatives are psyllium husks (can be sprinkled onto cereals or added to juices or smoothies) and flaxseeds (can be sprinkled onto cereals or added to salads). Flaxseeds have the added bonus of providing essential fatty acids as they are high in natural omega oils.

In other cases, herbal laxatives of varying strengths that increase gut motility can be used. Again, the use of laxatives is not the long-term solution to weight loss but in the short-term in conjunction with good nutrition and exercise, it will stimulate a sluggish digestive system and detoxify the blood of waste and prevent accumulation of toxins. The build up of toxins poses a number of health consequences which is never a good thing. Common herbal laxatives of decreasing strength that stimulate bowel movements include senna, butternut, rhubarb, yellow dock and dandelion root. It is highly recommended that a consultation with a medical herbalist is sought prior to self-medication as dosage and choice of herb requires specialist advice given within a holistic context.

- **Diuretics**

Many of the commercial brands for dieting (prepared either as teas, pills or tinctures) invariably have one or more herbal diuretics. Water retention is a real problem for some but many do not realise that poor dietary habits have probably led to that situation in the first place. In the short-term, it can be of benefit to the very few who have genuine water retention problems. However, for the vast majority diuretics have limited long-term value and only tricks the body into thinking it has lost weight when all it has achieved is to shed a few pounds of water. Diuretics can be addictive and can deplete the body of important nutrients and electrolytes such as sodium and potassium. In a strange paradoxical way, the best way to remedy the problem of water retention is to drink plenty of purified water as this will flush out the toxins that cause the retention of water in the first place. A lack of water causes the body to retain as much water as possible in as much as crash dieting and not eating very much in order to lose weight will trigger the body to go into 'starvation mode'. Therefore fat is retained much more as the body responds to a lack of food and prepares itself for a lengthy stint of starvation by holding onto its energy reserves (fat stores). Water is an essential component of our diet and though not strictly classified as a nutrient, we are dependent on it for our survival. Water is essential to keep us hydrated and to ensure that all our body systems work efficiently. This will prevent toxic build up which is the cause of so many illnesses and poor health. Effective herbal diuretics include dandelion, nettle and celery amongst others. It is strongly recommended that a consultation with a medical herbalist is sought prior to self-medication because a proper assessment of water retention can be made and a more effective weight loss programme can be devised which is specific to each person, their constitution and their lifestyle.

- **Appetite suppressants**

One of the biggest problems that dieters have is controlling hunger. Part of the strategy for weight loss has been in tackling this very problem. Appetite suppressants are now quite common in tackling obesity even in conventional medicine and last year alone, doctors in the UK issued over 1 million prescriptions for conventional anti-obesity drugs, such as sibutramine (marketed as Meridia® in the US and as Reductil® in Europe) and phentermine (marketed under various names). Other obesity drugs work by providing a sensation of fullness (satiation) by releasing 'feel good' chemicals from the brain similar to the feeling experienced by having a meal to quell hunger. Another popular drug that is prescribed is orlistat (marketed as Xenical® and Alli®) which works by preventing the absorption of fats from food, thereby reducing <u>calorie</u> intake. It is intended for use in conjunction with a calorie-controlled diet supervised by a doctor despite the fact that both are available OTC and impossible to monitor or supervise. Unfortunately, most or all of these anti-obesity drugs present some form of serious side effects and health risks such as heart complications, high blood pressure, nervous system problems and a host of mental health problems. It is hard to accept the judgement call for these prescriptions which in some areas have been given a greater financial priority over anti-cancer drugs or Alzheimer's drugs given that obesity is largely preventable.

It is somewhat unsurprising therefore that the natural plant substance extracted from the plant *hoodia gordonii* and marketed simply as hoodia (in various formulations and preparations) has widespread appeal as a natural appetite suppressant and has had much press attention. Traditionally, this is used by the San tribe bushmen of the Kalahari desert who consume only the inner portion and drink the white latex to suppress hunger whenever out on their long hunting expeditions. Research has revealed that the active constituent in this plant responsible for appetite suppression is a substance labelled as P57 and so far only one company has the exclusive rights to develop and market this active ingredient. Given this, it is surprising how many commercial brands of hoodia extract are available and freely marketed. Nevertheless, the only clinical trial (results of which are yet to be published) shows promise and so far, there have been no reported adverse effects from taking this herbs. However, it is important to buy the right product of reputable quality and whilst many of the brands are sold as whole plant preparations others have been found to have very little of the specific species of hoodia, being mixed with other varieties and worse still, synthetic ingredients which may pose health risks due to it being unregulated and unlicensed for sale. Many of the commercial brands through unregulated outlets have not been properly tested for safety and can prove risky to health.

It is highly recommended that a consultation with a medical herbalist is sought prior to purchase or self-medication. Proper advice and information on individual herbal remedies and preparations is vital in order to prevent the health consequences of taking unlicensed and unregulated commercial products.

Summary

In a climate of a global obesity crisis, it is becoming clear that many countries are facing a significant health problem for the future. This may have arisen for a number of reasons. Some of these are listed below:

- years of neglect through poor education and poor understanding of nutrition and food preparation
- irresponsible regulation and laws governing food manufacturing
- poor rearing of animals used for meat production
- increased use of hormones and other synthetic chemicals in food manufacturing
- increased availability of convenience and processed foods
- poor food labelling,
- increased food productivity
- increased sedentary lifestyles
- increased availability of cheap foods
- increased outlets for fast foods
- limited activity choices and affordability of sporting activities for young people
- low priority of physical education & sporting activities in schools
- poor nutritional content of school dinners

The above list is by no means an exhaustive list but it does give some indication of how the situation of obesity has become such a public health issue. To address this in any effective manner is going to require the efforts of government, health organisations, schools, employers and individuals. Effective policy, legislative enforcement in addition to a fundamental shift in attitude and culture about food is the only long-term solution to eradicate the many health consequences of obesity.

Increasing incidence of food allergies & food intolerence
The incidence of food allergies and food intolerances are on the increase and very much a big topic for discussion with nutritionists and health care practitioners. A leading UK charity, Allergy UK estimates that almost half of us have a sensitivity to certain foods, with over a million having a food allergy. 1 in 4 in the UK experiences an immediate and sometimes violent reaction ranging from an itchy rash to vomiting and abdominal pain. They also estimate that even greater numbers in the population have a food intolerance.

Food allergy is very different to food intolerance. Essentially, food allergy is an abnormal immune response in which an individual's immune system overreacts to foods that are ordinarily harmless. Antibodies produced attack the trigger substance in food and this starts a chain reaction of chemical changes which cause swelling and irritation in certain parts of the body affecting one or several organs or systems such as the skin, tongue and lips. Allergic reactions to food may threfore cause nausea, abdominal cramps or diarrhoea, sneezing or coughing. It may also result in a swollen tongue, lips or throat, tingling in the throat, tongue, lips or face, and very often produce hives or skin inflammations. Respiratory difficulties may arise due to tightness in the chest, shortness of breath or wheezing. It may also trigger an acute episode in asthmatics. The most dangerous allergic reaction is of course the anaphylactic shock (life-threatening respiratory distress). Therefore, susceptible individuals who have known food allergies, must avoid all foods containing the trigger substance.

Food intolerance on the other hand, is a physical reaction to a food or food additive that does not involve the immune system and commonly produces symptoms such as constipation, bloating and diarrhoea. Energy levels are low, accompanied by fatigue which could be exacerbated by a poor sleep pattern and resulting mood swings. There may also be outbreaks of eczema, thrush, headaches, frequent coughs and colds. Individuals who persistently suffer these symptoms on a regular basis probably haven't attributed these conditions to their diet. Rarely would people consider that what they eat could be making them ill and so for many, food intolerances go undetected for many years. Common examples of food intolerances include flavour enhancers such as monosodium glutamate (MSG) or preservatives such as sulphates. Other notable culprits include tyramine (a common food substance) found in a variety of foods such as cheese, caffeine in coffee, sulphites in wine, and phenylethylamine in chocolate. Milk intolerance is common particularly in cases of lactase enzyme deficiency which has a genetic basis. Food hypersensitivity reactions are usually associated with ingestion of chemicals added to or sprayed onto foods. Herbicides, pesticides (insecticides, fungicides for eg.), natural gas residues, antimicrobials, antibiotics, hormones, artificial flavourings and colourings, texture modifiers and packaging plastics are all examples of food and water contaminants that can trigger a host of hypersensitivity reactions in susceptible individuals. Given that food manufacturing and the very nature of food itself has changed considerably over the years, it is unsurprising that the incidence of food allergies and intolerances are as high as they are. If there is a dietary cause to symptoms, it is important to establish this as there can be a host of medical conditions and long-term health problems that are a direct result of adverse reactions to foods. Some examples are listed below:

- Sinus problems
- Glue ear
- IBS
- Abdominal bloating
- Constipation & diarrhoea
- Eczema
- Dermatitis
- Depression
- Panic attacks & anxiety
- Joint symptoms
- Heart problems & cardiovascular disease

Herbs that can be useful in dealing with symptoms of allergy have been discussed in Chapter 4 (under Allergies).

A consultation with a medical herbalist or a nutritionist is highly recommended so that any possible food allergies or intolerances can be identified. This may help with some of the symptoms which are difficult to understand and link to any single cause. A diet plan can be devised that includes suitable alternatives in cases of allergy and intolerance that does not compromise nutrition through eliminating certain foods from the diet.

Increasing incidence of infertility

Infertility has increased over the past 30 years with 1 in 4 couples being unable to conceive naturally. The increase in IVF treatments has given us one of the greatest indicators that infertility is on the increase. There may be a number of reasons for this including social changes and women having more choices so choosing to have children later in life and concentrating on their careers for longer. Of course fertility declines with age so trying to conceive later in life is that much more difficult. Moreover, the increasing incidence of sexually transmitted infections (STIs) means that scarring from repeated infection could lead to further increases in infertility. Other factors include physiological reasons such as endometriosis, polycystic ovarian syndrome (PCOS), low sperm count and blocked fallopian tubes. However, the majority of the causes are unexplained, that is, no structural or functional malfunction can be detected. This may mean that there is more than one cause to the infertility but importantly, it is the cue for us to look deeper at the underlying issues such as lifestyle factors, nutrition and emotional issues because addressing such fundamental and natural issues has proved incredibly successful. Therefore, it is clear that fertility itself is multi-factorial and a more holistic approach to tackling infertility is the only effective way forward in examining this worrying increase in our society today.

Stress and modern lifestyle means that little time is given to concentrating on building and strengthening relationships, time spent together, physically exhausted to have sex (frequency of sex should increase the chances), stress effects (this has a serious detrimental impact on reproductive function as well as libido) and poor nutrition (it is important to feed the body as this will enhance healthy development and production of both sperm and eggs).

The following gives some general advice on nutrition and lifestyle which has shown to improve the chances of conception. It is important to emphasise that the health of both the man and woman is equally important in fertility.

Nutritional changes:

In many cases, poor nutrition has had an influence on fertility. There are many foods commonly indicated to increase fertility although it is without doubt that a general, well-balanced healthy diet is always advised as this will ensure the healthy working of the reproductive systems in both men and women.

Common foods recommended for increasing fertility:

- **Folic Acid**. Folic acid is an important nutrient required for normal growth and reproduction. Deficiencies have been associated with serious birth defects, with a certain type of anaemia and with an increased risk of some types of cancers. It is vital to reproductive health to prevent a variety of birth defects including spina bifida. It can be found in leafy greens such as broccoli and lettuce

- **Iron**. Iron is required for energy production and deficiencies have been linked to problems with ovulation, a major factor in infertility. Iron-rich foods include lentils, soy beans and spinach

- **Calcium**. Calcium is required for the development of healthy bones and teeth, particularly for the growing baby. Important to your health and also helps the proper development of healthy bones and teeth in a developing fetus. Good sources of calcium include dairy products, greens and turnip

- **Zinc**. Zinc is required for healthy immune function, healthy skin and healthy sexual function. Deficiency in men leads to reduced testosterone levels which can impair sperm production but is also important in the healthy production of eggs. Good sources include asparagus, oysters, wheat germ, miso, lamb and summer squash

- **Fibre**. Fibre is needed to eliminate a variety of toxins from the body, thereby increasing your chances of getting pregnant. Foods that are excellent sources of fibre include beans and collard greens

- **Unsaturated Fats**. These healthy fats are good for a number of functions especially the immune system. Good sources include extra virgin olive oil, canola oil, fish and flax seed oil

- **Water**. Water flushes toxins from the body, which boosts fertility

Foods to Avoid:

- **Foods High in Saturated, Hydrogenated or Trans Fats**. Foods high in these fats increase the risk of being overweight or obese which limits fertility. There are also a host of other reasons why these fats should be avoided including the risk of hypertension which reduces male fertility. Foods high in these fats include fast foods, take away foods, processed foods and snacks.

- **White Flour**. Eating too much white flour can lead to constipation and this limits the removal of toxins from the body, thereby reducing fertility. Switch to whole grains which promote digestive system function and which can therefore improve fertility

- **Caffeine**. Caffeine has been linked to decreased fertility as with many of the stimulants. Limit or avoid caffeine-containing drinks and foods.

- **Alcohol**. Alcohol reduces fertility in both men and women by affecting various physiological mechanisms that are necessary for healthy reproductive function. If pregnant, and despite conflicting advice given by the medical professionals, it is best to avoid alcohol altogether. This will reduce the risk of birth defects and low birth weight.

- **Fad Diets**. It is never a good idea to diet especially using fad diets if trying to conceive. It is always best to eat healthily by having well-balanced meals in order to improve fertility.

It is also important to remember that a healthy diet goes hand-in-hand with regular, moderate exercise. Being either underweight or overweight can also reduce your fertility. An irregular Body Mass Index (BMI) can lead to infertility by causing irregular ovulation and menstrual cycles.

Lifestyle changes:
Cutting down or eliminating alcohol, giving up smoking, maintaining a healthy body weight (BMI needs to be between 18.5-24.9), taking adequate exercise and having plenty of rest & relaxation time/activities.

Combat stress:
One of the best ways to combat stress is to exercise. This needs to be aerobic exercise which means that the heart and lungs really get to work and ensure that blood reaches all the vital organs and tissues. Exercise has a host of benefits and is a general tonic for boosting libido, tackling stress, regulating weight, improving mental health, well-being and vitality.

Practical steps:
This includes making enough time to focus on the relationship, spending time together, building on the relationship and each other. Very often, couples are driven to regard the process of making a baby as a routine, functional process and this can make the entire process mechanical and lacking in emotion. Focusing on the romantic side of a relationship, the emotional well-being of each other can instigate passion and desire, a necessary prerequisite for increased frequency in having sex. The frequency is very important in fertility and many couples forget the art of romance and passion in their desperate desire to have a baby which has consumed all their emotional energy and left very little to concentrate on each other. It is best to also examine the reasons for having a baby and whether it will cement a relationship and it is what both want rather than fulfilling a 'tick-box' mentality.

Herbs are usually prescribed for specific problems such as erectile dysfunction or to regulate hormones. Disorders and problems that affect fertility have been discussed in detail in Chapter 4 (Herbal Healing). For specific problems and help, a consultation with a medical herbalist is recommended and may require referral to a specialist via the doctor/GP.

Mental health & herbal medicine
There is no question that mental health problems of the Western world are on the increase and given the stresses and strains of modern living, the statistics are unsurprising. A leading mental health charity in the

UK estimates that the current incidence of mental health problems is 1 in 4 soon to be 1 in 3. This includes problems such as depression, anxiety, eating disorders, dementia, personality disorder, obsessive compulsive disorder (OCD) and various others. Given the breakdown in family unit and the fact that many are left unsupported by society, merely left to 'get on with life' despite facing extreme difficulties, it is not surprising that people experience great mental distress and physical breakdown. Many of the drugs that are too easily prescribed often compound the problem and with complex conditions such as depression, it has been argued that prescription drugs do more harm than good.

It is clear that much of the problem of mental health in our society is in the way we live and the shifting values that place a huge burden on material gain equating success and happiness with material possessions and wealth. This is not assisted by the lack of emphasis on the spiritual health of the nation. The help available to support vulnerable people and those facing hardship is also dwindling so much so that a large part of the help is dependent on charities and volunteer groups. Many patients have reported that the NHS and the national health providers do not provide a suitable environment for healing since many are facing fear, loneliness and sometimes violence or sexual abuse in some of the hospital wards.

It is argued that the situation is getting worse due to the move to treat more people in the community and this means that it is only the most acute and distressed cases which are treated on wards. Mental illness can make people violent and paranoid, which is why some attacks happen. And mixed sex wards, which are still relatively common, make things worse. Some wards are dirty, depressing and dangerous. This is no way to help people in recovery from mental health problems. And it does not need to be like this – we are talking about one of the most vulnerable groups within society.

Sadly, mental illness continues to be stigmatised both in society and in the workplace with employers giving little regard and support for sufferers to either get back into the workplace or to receive the specific help for them to get better. Much of the work of CAM healthcare practitioners such as medical herbalists is to provide the much needed support for sufferers of mental illness and to campaign for better services and specialist help including talking therapies, self-help groups and possibly medical help for those affected. Herbal medicines themselves provide much-needed assistance through a range of nervines and tonics which are individually tailored for each patient. This can help with the wide variety of symptoms that are common and specific formulations can be of immense value in many of the mental health conditions so frequent in modern societies today. Useful herbs include the following:

- **St. John's Wort** – mild to moderate depression, anxiety
- **Skullcap** – nerve tonic, sedative, nervous tension
- **Wood betony** – sedative, nerve tonic, nervous exhaustion, anxiety
- **Damiana** – nerve tonic, stimulant, antidepressant, useful in nervous debility
- **Chamomile** – relaxant, sedative, extremely useful in anxiety and nervous tension
- **Hops** – hypnotic, sedative, good for sleep disorders
- **Oats** – nerve tonic, nutrient, good for nervous debility
- **Vervain** – nerve tonic, good for depression and nervous exhaustion
- **Valerian** – good for sleep disorders and anxiety states
- **Ginsengs** – extremely useful in stress-related disorders, anxiety and nervous exhaustion

Organisations aim to establish effective links with external agencies, lobbyists and the NHS to improve services and networks for information delivery and education on mental health and its various complexities that affect a great many people in society today.

Natural alternatives to antibiotics

The current concern regarding hospital-acquired infections (HAIs) has prompted a review on the use or more appropriately perhaps, the overuse of antibiotics, the politically-charged issue of hospital cleanliness and our general immune defences. Infections such as MRSA (methicillin-resistant *Staphylococcus aureus*), *Clostridium difficile* and more recent VRSA (vancomycin-resistant *Staphylococcus aureus*) are a real concern for hospitals and healthcare practitioners. However it is not relevant here to discuss in detail the reasons why HAIs have become a major item on the NHS agenda.

Many of the historical debates on this subject have focussed on the overuse of antibiotics and the development of antibiotic resistance in patients who then become susceptible to HAIs. Much time and funds have been invested in changing the prescription protocol and attitudes to antibiotics which by and large, through long-term use can weaken a natural immune system and increase the body's risk to 'superbugs', the more virulent or stronger strain of infectious agents.

Natural alternatives to antibiotics have always been around and are gaining more prominence because it has a greater appeal to those who are concerned about antibiotic overuse and those who want to promote a healthier approach to boosting their immune defences, health and vitality. To a large extent, physicians are trained to prescribe medicines but arguably, where it has gone wrong is in the frequency with which antibiotics are used, in particular as a preventative measure or in minor infections such as sore throat there is an unhealthy abundance of it in many of our foods, OTC medicines and toiletries so it is unsurprising that infectious agents have developed a resistance to it by mutating to form stronger, tougher versions of their original self.

There are a number of ways to adopt a more natural approach to improving resistance to infection. This is both curative and preventative and therefore the preferred choice for many people worried about antibiotic overuse. The use of herbal supplements (immune enhancers, immune boosters, herbal antibiotics and vitamin/mineral supplementation) will also prevent the recurrence of infection. Parents who are worried about their children being prescribed antibiotics especially their side effects may wish to consider these alternatives particularly since children respond extremely well to herbal remedies and it is where I have seen many of the best examples of natural approaches work very well indeed. Some common examples of natural alternatives include the following:

Herbal immune boosters and anti-infective herbs:

Ginsengs

Wild indigo

Echinacea

Tree of life

Tea tree oil

Goldenseal

Clove oil

Eucalyptus oil

Myrrh

Culinary herbs, spices and foods:

Garlic

Ginger

Turmeric

Basil

Honey

Cayenne

General supplements:

Vitamins A, C and E

Zinc

L-Arginine

Grapeseed extract

For specific help on herbal medicines, nutrition and supplementation to boost immune defences, to fight infection and to prevent recurrent infections, a consultation with a medical herbalist is highly recommended.

(ii) Toxicity issues & recent scare stories

Much has been written about herbs and whilst some are highly favourable reports on their usefulness in a range of medical conditions and disorders, some reports are extremely misleading, incomplete, inadequately researched and based on very little scientific data merely on evidential reporting and anecdotal findings. This has unsurprisingly caused some concern with the discerning consumer who may be alarmed at the toxicity issues surrounding some herbs and worried about potential damage to their health.

It is to be accepted that the scientific community and the medical profession will always be concerned about patient safety as a priority as do so many other health care professionals including medical herbalists. Whilst some scientists are careful observers and objective with their analysis, others appear hell bent on discrediting herbal medicine. It would be interesting to see the declared interests when it comes to funding such studies.

With many of the popular herbs so readily available from non-reputable and unregulated sources, the risks of buying a product that has not been tested for safety raises some worrying questions. Online shopping has by far caused the greatest concern since the sources of the herbs cannot be verified and whilst it is illegal for any UK supplier to sell any unlicensed and untested products on the market (online or through standard retail outlets) it is not illegal for any UK citizen to buy any such illegal products from the internet. Therefore, it remains the responsibility of health care practitioners, consumer groups, patient groups and other similar interested parties to educate and inform on the dangers of unlicensed and unregulated products. The regulatory authorities who act as watchdog for such illegal practices; the Medicines & Healthcare Products

Regulatory Agency (MHRA) and the Foods Standards Agency (FSA) in the UK and the Food & Drugs Administration (FDA) in the US have some power to control and regulate such illegal practices although this does not necessarily safeguard the public who are swayed by powerful advertising and marketing of unlicensed online products.

Unfortunately, those rare cases of toxicity and adverse effects have had a detrimental impact on the image of herbal medicine and have tarnished its reputation. This has generated some controversy whether herbs are in fact safe let alone effective. Due to the potency of some herbal remedies, only qualified and registered practitioners of herbal medicine are permitted to dispense some herbs whilst others, though readily available are best taken through individually tailored prescriptions and following proper advice and guidance from practitioners.

Kava kava For anxiety. Banned in Britain because of three deaths and six transplants resulting from liver toxicity. The oldest professional body for medical herbalists have campaigned vigorously for its reinstatement because it was found that patients already had impaired liver function and the herb should not have been indicated. The benefits of kava far outweighs any risks that have arisen through poor prescription practices in compromised patients.

Ginkgo biloba prescribed for a host of dementia-related disorders as well as for improving circulation. Some concern over possible increased risk of brain haemorrhage and stroke but this has not been proven. Interactions with antiplatelets drugs so self-adminstration is not advisable.

Devil's claw prescribed for arthritic pain and inflammation. Some gastric symptoms because it may increase stomach acid and so should be avoided by people with ulcers. However, the herb can be administered as enteric coated capsules or tablets which will limit acid production whilst also protecting the active ingredients of the herb from stomach acid interaction.

Saw palmetto prescribed for enlarged prostate. Should not be taken with drugs like aspirin or warfarin which increase bleeding

St John's Wort prescribed for mild to moderate depression with favourable scientific proof of effectiveness. However, it has a host of interactions with other drugs (xref Chapter 3 – top 20 herbs). Depression requires proper diagnosis and management so it is strongly recommended that advice is sought prior to self-medication as a referral in serious cases may be required for effective treatment.

Valerian prescribed for insomnia. Dosage considerations are important as it can produce a drowziness similar to a hangover at high doses. Best to consult a herbalist before self-medication.

Hawthorn prescribed for congestive heart disease which is too serious a condition for self-medication. Indiscriminate administration is not recommended for such cases.

Willow bark prescribed for pain relief but should not be taken if asthmatic or in patients who have gastric ulcers. Strongly advisable that a consultation with a herbalist is sought prior to self-medication

Echinacea works best as a prophylactic against the common cold. Some people have allergic reactions. This is very rare and again, the benefits of the herb far outweigh any adverse effect.

Whilst it is acknowledged that herbs are effective medicines, it is without doubt that taking unlicensed and unregulated products through non-reputable sources or those not prescribed by a medical herbalist can have significant adverse effects which can include toxicity. Many of the herbs have drug interactions (problems of which are described below) and so caution should be advised, particularly if self-medicating. However, there is much to be gained from herbal medicines and irresponsible reporting can be alarmist which is not only unnecessary but limits consumer choice and focuses entirely on evidence-based drugs prescribed only by doctors. The benefits of herbs properly dispensed and administered far outweigh any of the scare stories that are reported through misinformation and as a result of taking unregulated and unlicensed products. One can only wonder if the unrelenting campaign to discredit natural medicines is instigated by some edict to pursue a case against consumer choice or because herbal medicines by their very nature can have no involvement or vested interest from the global pharmaceutical industries.

(iii) Herb-drug interactions

Before Western Herbal Medicine achieved its present popularity, particularly in the UK and US, the need for raising concern over possible interactions between herbs and prescription drugs was not as pressing as in recent years. Any possible cases of adverse reactions or interactions were confined to isolated incidents and probably attributed to errors in dosing, inappropriate administration and poor patient education of concomitant use. It appears that little has changed. However, a lack of evidential reporting of this nature does not preclude its existence and to ascertain the true number of cases or indeed the first incident of herb-drug interaction has proved extremely difficult.

Awareness of potential risks of herb-drug interactions remains poor particularly as clinical monitoring of herbal prescriptions is not as rigorous as conventional medicines. In more recent years, this has been addressed through a system comparable to conventional medicine and so it has become easier to monitor herb-drug interactions. Moreover, conducting clinical audits of herbal medical practice is rendered inaccurate and invalid especially when concentrations of active constituents (AC) can vary significantly according to brand, preparation, harvesting and processing. Difficulties in this area will therefore persist and may prove entirely irrelevant to herbal medicine. This poses additional problems in establishing potential risks of concomitant administration. A lack of standardisation in herbal medicine preparations leads to variable concentrations of AC that can be accounted for but also renders it difficult to ensure parity of product quality, especially in light of a competitive and brutal commercial market.

In as much as a clinical audit is nigh on impossible under such parameters, so too is the prediction of possible adverse interactions with prescription drugs. Recent debates over legislative enforcement in regulating herbal medicine in Britain, has clearly highlighted opportunities for research that ought to be exploited without delay. Herb-drug interaction is a serious issue that requires funding for extensive and immediate study. However, would Statutory Self Regulation (SSR) necessarily prompt rigorous scientific study into potential and established interactions if scientific credibility of herbal medicine is yet to be proved and whilst orthodox scientists remain sceptical of the efficacy of herbal remedies?

With the widespread availability of herbal remedies within the public domain, it is quite surprising that the issue of herb-drug interaction has not surfaced sooner. It is clear however, that the urgency for education and action is gathering momentum and as information about drugs continues to increase exponentially, the number of reported drug interactions parallels this increase. Over the last few years some foodstuffs, most notably grapefruit juice, have also attracted attention as causing a possible adverse interaction with drugs. Herb-drug interactions present serious concerns in the clinical setting and warrant much discussion, particularly in a current climate of increased availability of herbal remedies and over-prescription of conventional drugs. Unequivocally, the newer brands of pharmacological agents that have higher potency and side effects pose fresh challenges and opportunities for study in this area of medicine. Reported cases of adverse interactions must be viewed as individual cases but equally, it must set a precedent for a prescription protocol based on known and proven biochemical basis for risk. Moreover, it should instigate a thorough review for screening established and potential basis for herb-drug interaction for all medicinal herbs commonly prescribed by herbalists.

Without doubt, public perception of herbal remedies as safe, at any dose, and the fact that patients do not always inform their GPs/doctors of concomitant use has to change. This requires a coordinated effort involving education, dissemination of proper information and implementation, which in all likelihood can ensure some measure in safe practice at all levels of the therapeutic process. Unfortunately, a lack of legislative protection and scientific credibility is such that it is the herbal medicine profession that is scrutinised more thoroughly in cases of adverse interactions and invariably in an unfavourable light. Current literature on the subject is significant but by no means extensive in respect of being comparable to orthodox drug reviews. However, the data can prove useful in exercising caution and setting a prescription protocol in susceptible or high risk groups such as the elderly. A critique of clinical trials on herbs has clearly highlighted that research needs to be more rigorous and robust in terms of scientific validity, especially if it is to be regarded as a true comparable to orthodox drug trials.

It is evident that practitioners of both forms of medicine require training and updates on this aspect of practice, in addition to the mutual sharing of information, since both professions, in respect of herb-drug interaction impact on each other. The prospect of working more closely with regulatory authorities and offering the public a vital service in ensuring safety when taking herbal medicines, also means that herbal medical practice and the work of pharmacologists have become interdependent. This ought to establish a forum for research and communication between the two professions; herbal practitioners routinely treat patients who are taking conventional drugs and it is essential that they have reliable information about possible interactions.

Additionally, the role of the herbal medicine practitioner is absolutely vital in risk assessment and risk counselling. Examining all reported cases of interactions could be compiled for investigation; this may confirm the biochemical basis for risk or highlight susceptibility in certain clinical presentations. Further investigation is also required and although fundamentally, the synergy of AC in herbal preparations dictates the crucial effective tool in therapy, it is theoretically possible that such AC could cause adverse interactions or sensitivities in predisposed individuals.

(iv) Availability & popularity of herbal supplements

As highlighted above, the availability and popularity of herbal supplements means that it is subject to unscrupulous manufacturers and persuasive advertising. From the consumer's perspective, there is a bewildering array of choices and choosing the brand, herb, dosage and preparation type is particularly difficult. This is why I always advise people to consult a medical herbalist first before self-medicating. Many of the market brands available in retail outlets and health food shops may not necessarily be harmful as the stringent controls mean that they are subjected to quality control prior to being sold over the counter. This should test for any unwanted products or worse still, toxic substances. However, it does not guarantee the effectiveness of some of the brands since they can vary significantly and at best they may be safe but may not be particularly effective as they may contain very little active herbal ingredients.

I normally tell those who ask that it is never recommended that they buy a local or chain supermarket brand, nor any of the high street chemists' brand or the own brands from chain health food shops. The quality is not always great and many are persuaded by the cheap deals or bulk buys. On a long-term basis, this is not sensible and it is far more cost-effective to spend a little more on a brand of better quality which is likely to be effective rather than wasting money on supplements which are no better than chalk tablets.

Online purchasing is a mixed bag.... if you know the brand and it has been recommended, it is safe to purchase them but ONLY from their own brand's website if you want to be totally safe. However, there are other outlets that will sell these recommended brands so it may be worthwhile spending some time investigating the best option for you. It always astonishes me that so many are incredibly careless about what they purchase as supplements online without any regard to its safety or quality. They may as well be swallowing a whole load of placebos but worse still, it is hard to tell whether any of the products have any dangerous substances in them. Some of the unknown brands may have sub-therapeutic doses or may contain added ingredients (for example bulking agents, excipients or adjuvants) that are not listed in the ingredients. It is this very sort of thing that can prove to be unsafe as it is impossible to trace the cause of any adverse reaction or side effect to the supplement. The guarantee and reassurance that one has when purchasing from the brand's own website is really in its safety and effectiveness. A reputable high street health food shop (usually NOT part of a chain) should stock a good range of the above-mentioned brands. These shops normally sell whole foods and a range of other health products so it is worth investigating your nearest store.

Many people are keen to explore herbal alternatives and supplements to improve their health or to tackle the symptoms of a current condition. However, they may not always know the best herb to take and the preparation type. My advice in cases of uncertainty is to consult a medical herbalist as they are trained to help with this very type of question and to work out the best form of treatment as well as preparation type (eg. tablets vs tinctures etc...).

FAQ include:
- Which brand is the best one?
- Is the product I buy of good quality?

- Does my brand contain the correct quantity of active constituents?
- Why do brands vary so much in their effectiveness?
- What about the sources of the herbs?
- Is the product ethically sourced and produced?

This book, in part goes some way towards answering some of these questions and providing some basic information on this very aspect of consumer concerns. However, for specific help on a current or ongoing health condition, it is strongly recommended that a consultation with a qualified and registered practitioner of herbal medicine is sought. They will be able to answer specific questions about some of the more popular commercial brands and make recommendations about future purchases of OTC herbal supplements.

CHAPTER 7 – CONCLUSIONS

(i)   The future of healthcare
(ii)   The contribution of Western herbal medicine to healthcare

(i) The future of healthcare

Many advances have been made in modern medicine and conventional healthcare practices. Despite this, there continues to be a growing demand for natural therapies and alternatives to modern medicine. Whilst there is a place for both forms of healthcare, an ideal future would encompass both systems that offer patients a greater choice of treatments and therapies that yields the best clinical outcomes. A truly integrated system of healthcare will focus on health and healing rather than mere disease and treatment. Its mission is to involve other treatments, therapies and modalities, often CAM therapies in order to treat the many diseases of modern society today. To achieve this, there has to be much liaison between conventional doctors and practitioners of other disciplines which necessitates the sharing of vital information and the exchange of ideas and concepts in the healing process. There are also differing perspectives of various countries that give rise to differing medical practices with varying levels of integration between conventional medicine and traditional practices such as herbal medicine.

Integrative medicine views patients as whole people with minds and spirits as well as bodies and there is much emphasis on lifestyle, diet, rest, sleep and relationships. The recent reports on the ineffectiveness of conventional antidepressants in mild to moderate depression is yet another example of why a holistic approach is much needed to treat the many conditions of modern living.

The holistic approach to diagnosis and treatment has a very real place in modern medicine today despite some of its limitations. A truly integrated approach involving other modalities and therapies must take into account the constitutional differences of patients and will require much cooperation, effort and support from medical organisations, government, patient groups and individuals. The successful future of healthcare lies in this very approach and the contributions of CAM such as herbal medicine is immense, particularly in addressing many of the chronic illnesses witnessed within modern societies today.

(ii) The contribution of Western herbal medicine to healthcare

Western herbal medicine has much to offer by way of healthcare in modern life. Not only is it immensely useful in treating a variety of symptoms in a range of illnesses and chronic disease, it is also a valuable addition to the whole process of preventative medicine which considers aspects of nutrition and lifestyle amongst other factors which predispose to illness.

The work of medical herbalists not only covers the integral issues of diagnosis and treatment but also explores broader aspects of spirituality, the mind-body link, understanding of the self, identity and harmony with our environment, living as a community, all of which is sadly lacking in some manner or form in modern society today.

Western herbal medicine offers natural alternatives and a greater patient choice for those who are dissatisfied with modern drug therapy and are concerned about side-effects or the long-term use of strong medicines. In its entirety, the holistic approach, the emphasis on individuals and the strong history and traditions provide a valuable foundation for modern herbal practice within clinical medicine. The contribution of Western herbal medicine is substantial and there is a determined effort from professional bodies, doctors, allied health professionals, CAM practitioners, patients groups and lobbyists to campaign for political change that legislates for an improved provision of CAM therapies within the national framework of healthcare services. This may take some time but remains a contentious debate in political circles, the medical profession and the scientific community.

RECOMMENDED READING & USEFUL ADDRESSES

Recommended Reading:
Saxelby, C. (2002). Nutrition for Life, everything you need to know about food and nutrition. Hardie Grant Books. ISBM 1-74064-014-4

Pitchford, P. (2002). Healing with whole foods. Asian traditions and modern nutrition. 3rd edition. North Atlantic Books. ISBN 1-55643-471-5

Williams, X. (1998). The herbal detox plan. The revolutionary way to cleanse and revive your body. Vermilion. London. ISBN 0-09187-672-9

Stoll, A.L. (2001). Omega-3 connection. How you can restore your mental well-being and beat memory loss and depression. Simon & Schuster. ISBN 0-7432-0709-2

Servan-Schreiber, D. (2004). Healing without Freud or Prozac. Natural approaches to curing stress, anxiety and depression without drugs and without psychoanalysis. Rodale, USA. ISBN 1-4050-6718-7

Murray, M. (1995). Stress, anxiety & insomnia. How you can benefit from diet, vitamins, minerals, herbs, exercise and other natural methods. Prima Publishing, USA. ISBN 1-559-489-0

McKenna, J. (2003). Natural alternatives to antibiotics. Newleaf. Dublin. ISBN 0-7171-3435-0

Professional Bodies & Finding a Practitioner:
The National Institute of Medical Herbalists (NIMH): www.nimh.org.uk
British Association of Nutritional Therapists (BANT): www.bant.org.uk
Institute of Optimum Nutrition (ION): www.ion.ac.uk
Federation o Holistic Therapists (FHT): www.fht.org.uk
College of Practitioners of Phytotherapists (CPP): www.phytotherapists.org
Institute for Complementary Medicine (ICM): www.i-c-m.org.uk
American Herbalists Guild (AHG): www.americanherbalistsguild.com

Useful Organisations:
MIND: National Association for Mental Health. Tel: 0845 766 0163. www.mind.org.uk
SANE: Mental Health Charity (UK) www.sane.org.uk
MHRA: Medicines and Healthcare Products Regulatory Agency www.mca.gov.uk/mhra/index.htm

Other useful contacts details:
FSA (Food Standards Agency): Tel: 0207 276 8000. www.eatwell.gov.uk
BHF (British Heart Foundation): Tel: 0845 070 8070. www.bhf.org.uk
Diabetes UK: Tel: 0845 120 2960. www.diabetes.org.uk
NHS Choices: www.nhs.uk
NHS Direct: Tel: 0845 4647. www.nhsdirect.nhs.uk

INDEX

Lightning Source UK Ltd.
Milton Keynes UK
19 February 2011

167826UK00002B/1/P

9 781609 106393